MAJOR PROBLEMS IN INTERNAL MEDICINE

Published

Cline: Cancer Chemotherapy (third edition by Cline and Haskell now available separately)
Shearn: Sjögren's Syndrome
Cogan: Ophthalmic Manifestations of Systemic Vascular Disease
Williams: Rheumatoid Arthritis as a Systemic Disease
Cluff, Caranasos and Stewart: Clinical Problems with Drugs
Fries and Holman: Systemic Lupus Erythematosus
Kass: Pernicious Anemia
Braude: Antimicrobial Drug Therapy
Bray: The Obese Patient
Zieve and Levin: Bleeding Disorders
Gorlin: Coronary Artery Disease
Bunn, Forget and Ranney: Hemoglobinopathies
Sleisenger and Brandborg: Malabsorption
Beeson and Bass: The Eosinophil
Krugman and Gocke: Viral Hepatitis
Hurwitz, Duranceau, and Haddad: Disorders of Esophageal Motility
Galambos: Cirrhosis
Nelson: The Adrenal Cortex: Physiological Function and Disease
Raskin and Appenzeller: Headache
Brooks: Disorders of the Exocrine Pancreas
Cupps and Fauci: The Vasculitides
Lieber: Medical Disorders of Alcoholism—Pathogenesis and Treatment
Scheinberg and Sternlieb: Wilson's Disease

MAJOR PROBLEMS IN INTERNAL MEDICINE

In Preparation

Kilbourne: Influenza
Weinstein: Infective Endocarditis

SARCOIDOSIS
and Other Granulomatous Disorders

WITHDRAWN

D. GERAINT JAMES, M.A., M.D., F.R.C.P., LL.D. (Hon.)

Senior Physician
Royal Northern Hospital
London, England

and

W. JONES WILLIAMS, M.D., F.R.C.P., F.R.C.Path.

University of Wales
College of Medicine
Department of Pathology
Llandough Hospital
Cardiff, Wales

Volume 24
in the series

MAJOR PROBLEMS IN INTERNAL MEDICINE

Lloyd H. Smith, Jr., M.D., *Editor*

1985
W. B. SAUNDERS COMPANY

Philadelphia □ London □ Toronto □ Mexico City □ Rio de Janeiro □ Sydney □ Tokyo

W. B. Saunders Company: West Washington Square
Philadelphia, PA   19105

1 St. Anne's Road
Eastbourne, East Sussex BN21 3UN, England

1 Goldthorne Avenue
Toronto, Ontario M8Z 5T9, Canada

Apartado 26370—Cedro 512
Mexico 4, D.F., Mexico

Rua Coronel Cabrita, 8
Sao Cristovao Caixa Postal 21176
Rio de Janeiro, Brazil

9 Waltham Street
Artarmon, N.S.W. 2064, Australia

Ichibancho, Central Bldg., 22-1 Ichibancho
Chiyoda-Ku, Tokyo 102, Japan

Library of Congress Cataloging in Publication Data

James, D. Geraint (David Geraint)

Sarcoidosis and other granulomatous disorders.

(Vol. 24 in the series Major problems in internal medicine)

1. Sarcoidosis.   2. Granuloma.   I. Williams, W. Jones
(William Jones)   II. Title.   III. Series: Major problems
in internal medicine; v. 24.   [DNLM: 1. Granuloma.   2.
Sarcoidosis.   W1 MA492T v.24/QZ 140 J27s]

RC182.S14J36 1985   616.99'3   84–22197

ISBN 0–7216–1044–7

Sarcoidosis and Other Granulomatous Disorders   ISBN 0–7216–1044–7

Last digit is the print number: 9   8   7   6   5   4   3   2   1

FOREWORD

In medicine, as in many other human pursuits, the obscure tends to fascinate. Perhaps this explains in part the deep interest that internists have long maintained in sarcoidosis, an interest disproportionate to the statistical role of this perplexing disorder in the spectrum of human illness. It beguiles us in yet another way; it is remarkably versatile in its clinical manifestations, intruding into innumerable differential diagnostic schema. The granulomas take up residence in a wide variety of organs and organ systems; in fact, all of them are at risk. As a result, the clinical presentation often represents a disordered mix of symptoms and dysfunctions in patterns that are difficult to categorize.

Yet many have tried to capture the disease and encase it in a neat nosology, buttressed by eponyms. Rarely have so many proper names from so many countries been used to encapulate fragments of an elusive entity: Hutchinson, Boeck, Besnier, Lofgren, Heerfordt, Schaumann, and even Mortimer (of malady fame). Over the years, the cause of sarcoidosis has been discovered many times to be various unusual organisms or to be the immune response to particular environmental factors in perceived sarcoid belts. But the mystery still remains, more than a century after Jonathan Hutchinson's description of the skin lesions in his gouty patient.

We should not conceive of sarcoidosis as simply a mass of inert nodules peppered randomly throughout various parts of the body to the discomfiture of the host. The lesion presumably represents some kind of immunological battlefield, to use Geraint James' phrase, with its own dynamics of attack and defense. No provocateur of this warfare (some presumed antigen of exogenous origin) has as yet been implicated in a reproducible manner. Attention has therefore been turned to the granulomatous process itself with its confusing interplay of monocytes, activated macrophages, epithelioid cells, giant cells, inclusion bodies, transformed T cells, activated B cells, and the various associated lymphokines. Progress in understanding granuloma formation clearly depends on the cell biology of the immune response itself.

Fortunately this is an area of intensive investigation and rapidly developing new insights.

This monograph, *Sarcoidosis and Other Granulomatous Disorders,* is an admirable summary of the field with an appropriate balance of clinical medicine and laboratory science. Drs. James and Jones Williams have had extensive experience with sarcoidosis—a series of over 800 patients during the past thirty years—so that this treatise carries the authority of sustained personal scholarship as well as a comparative review of world experience. We are therefore proud to include this monograph as the 24th book in the series *Major Problems in Internal Medicine.*

LLOYD H. SMITH, JR.

PREFACE

Sarcoidosis has been with us for 100 years or so; it needs to be updated every so often. In Sir Jonathan Hutchinson's days it was a dermatological curiosity, but in the twilight of his life radiography was introduced and it became a multisystem disorder. During this century sarcoidosis has been chased, like an overblown beach ball, by clinicians, pathologists, radiologists, chemists, chest physicians, ophthalmologists, gastro-enterologists, and, more recently, by epidemiologists, geneticists, and immunologists. Each fresh approach has added new dimensions. All these data must be brought together so that a unitarian concept of sarcoidosis and its many cousins with a similar pathology may emerge. More knowledge of the many other granulomatous disorders should help us to unravel the remaining enigma, namely, the aetiology of sarcoidosis.

This review presents data from our own series of 818 patients personally investigated and managed during the last 30 years in one weekly Sarcoidosis Clinic. This provides a homogenous viewpoint of the management of sarcoidosis. We have added international breadth and heterogeneity by comparing this series with a group of 3,676 patients studied in several different sarcoidosis clinics around the world. The data are surprisingly similar worldwide and also in Eastern Europe.

This update also includes studies derived from our attendance at and participation in ten international conferences on sarcoidosis and other granulomatous disorders (1958–1984).

This review, which includes 90 tables and 115 figures, is by one physician and one pathologist; our disciplines are diverse and complementary, but our love of sarcoidosis is singular.

If this monograph saves the sight of just one person, then it has been worthwhile.

D. GERAINT JAMES
W. JONES WILLIAMS

ACKNOWLEDGMENTS

This work was done within the structure of the British National Health Service, and it would have been much more difficult to accumulate all these solid data outside of it. We are also grateful to Friends of the Royal Northern Hospital, Roger Ghibbs, the E B Hutchinson Trust, and Tenovus. Many distinguished scientific journals have granted us permission to reproduce information already published—the Journal of the Royal College of Physicians; Annals of the New York Academy of Sciences; and the Journal of Clinical and Experimental Immunology.

Our ever-supportive wives, Sheila and Rosemary, do not want this volume to be dedicated to them. They prefer our salute to be directed to those who have gone before; their photographs are in Chapter 1.

CONTENTS

1
Historical Background 1
2
Descriptive Definition and Classification of Granulomatous Disorders 17
3
Pathology 21
4
Multisystem Clinical Features 38
5
Intrathoracic and Upper Respiratory Tract 49
6
Ocular and Neurosarcoidosis 77
7
The Skin 97
8
Sarcoidosis of the Heart 112
9
Lymphoreticular System 118
10
Locomotor System 132
11
Miscellaneous Involvement 144
12
Biochemistry 163
13
Immunology 174
14
Criteria of Activity 192
15
Differential Diagnosis 199
16
Aetiology 216

17
Treatment 222
   18
Epidemiology 233
Index 246

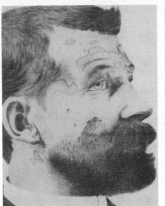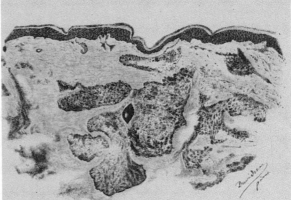

Figure 1–4

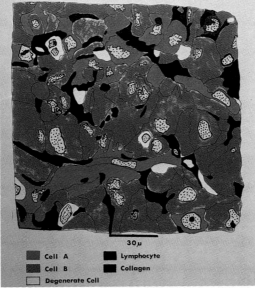

■ Cell A	■ Lymphocyte
■ Cell B	■ Collagen
□ Degenerate Cell	

30μ

Figure 3–5

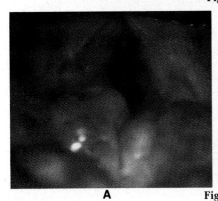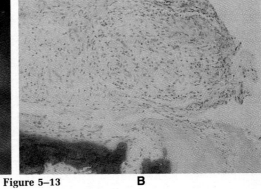

A   Figure 5–13   B

PLATE I

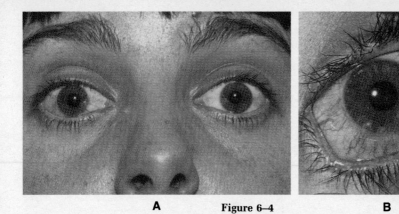

A   Figure 6–4   B

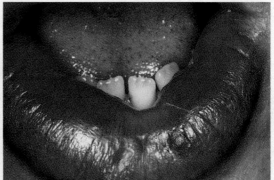

Figure 7–6   Figure 11–3

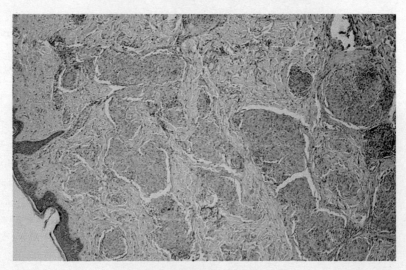

Figure 13–1

PLATE II

1

Historical Background

JONATHAN HUTCHINSON

In the years preceding and following the turn of the 19th century, several publications independently drew attention to what is now regarded as sarcoidosis. Depending on the authors' interests, the articles separately described skin lesions, bone cysts, parotid and eye involvement, and lymph-adenopathy. The diversity of tissues involved was matched only by the variety of synonyms invoked by the authors, who were unaware of the essential unity of the various manifestations of the disease. Furthermore, dermatologists themselves were uncertain whether their published examples were related to descriptions previously reported, and even illustrated, by others. In this way confusion grew, and both synonyms and eponyms multiplied to a score. The historical background well illustrates the protean clinical manifestations of sarcoidosis (Table 1–1).

The first recorded and illustrated example of sarcoidosis seen in the 19th century is attributed to Jonathan Hutchinson.[1] His patient, John W—— (Fig. 1–1), was a florid man of 58 years of age who worked at a coal wharf. He came under Hutchinson's care at the Blackfriars Hospital for Skin Diseases, London, in January 1869 and remained under his observation for one year. Hutchinson felt that the skin lesions were in some way related to the patient's gout.

He came on account of a number of peculiar patches of dark purplish colour on his extremities . . . He had an attack of gout in the metacarpo-phalangeal joint of his left forefinger while under treatment. No medicine had much effect on the eruption; he took at different times, colchicum and magnesia, arsenic, acid iron mixture, iodide of potassium, and simple alkaline mixture. No special local treatment was adopted, only an ointment of lead and mercury being ordered . . .

The facsimile (Fig. 1–2) is Hutchinson's first published account of this patient under the title "Case of livid papillary psoriasis," which appeared in his *Illustrations of Clinical Surgery* (1877).[1] In a much later publication "On eruptions which occur in connection with gout",[2] Hutchinson recalls this first example with the remark ". . . He had suffered from gout . . . "

John W——died in 1875 at the age of 64 years from kidney disease, following treatment at King's College Hospital, London. It is now recognized that patients with sarcoidosis occasionally have disordered calcium metabolism leading to renal calculi and terminal renal failure. It is interesting to

1

Table 1–1. Landmarks in the History of Sarcoidosis

Year	Landmark
1798–1808	Robert Willan's treatise "On Cutaneous Diseases" is published with a vivid description and copperplate engraving in colour of erythema nodosum.
1869	John W——, a florid 58-year-old coal-wharf worker, is attended by Jonathan Hutchinson at Hospital for Skin Diseases, London.
1875	John W— dies of renal failure, King's College Hospital, London.
1889	Caesar Boeck succeeds Carl Wilhelm Boeck and Bidenkap in charge of skin diseases, Christiania (Oslo).
	Besnier coins term *Lupus pernio*.
1892	Tenneson describes histology of lupus pernio.
1895	Jonathan Hutchinson presents Mrs. Mortimer to the London Dermatological Society. She refuses skin biopsy.
1897	Caesar Boeck presents to the Christiania Medical Society his 34-year-old police constable with skin lesions and lymphadenopathy, together with skin biopsy histology of sarcoid tissue.
1898	Osler—chronic lacrimal and parotid gland enlargement.
1902	Kienbock ⎤
1904	Kreibich ⎬ Bone changes
1910	Reider ⎟
1920	Jungling ⎦
1906	Darier and Roussy—Subcutaneous nodules
1909	Schumaker ⎤
	Heerfordt ⎬ Uveitis
1910	Bering ⎦
1915	Jorgen Schaumann—Zambaco Prise
	Kuznitsky and Bittorf—Chronic skin and pulmonary lesions
1935	Salvesen—Plasma protein elevation
1937	Bruins-Slot ⎤
	Longcope and Pierson ⎬ Uveoparotid fever
	Pautrier ⎟
	Waldenström ⎦
1935	Williams ⎤
1941	Kveim ⎟
1943	Danbolt ⎬ Kveim-Siltzbach test
	Putkonen ⎟
1949	Nelson ⎟
1954	Siltzbach ⎦
1946	Sven Löfgren's syndrome

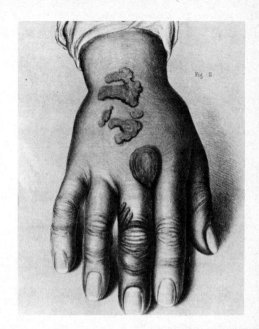

Figure 1–1. John W——.

speculate whether John W——'s skin lesions and terminal renal disease were interrelated.

THE BOECKS

In the summer of 1869, Hutchinson visited Christiania University, where Dr. Bidenkap showed him a collection of pathological drawings in the University Museum. Among these was one of a patient of Professor Carl Wilhelm Boeck (1808–75) illustrating skin lesions similar to those of John W—— on the hand of a healthy Swedish sailor who did not suffer from gout. Professor Boeck was an uncle of Caesar Boeck (1845–1917), who was later to make valuable contributions to the study of sarcoidosis. Both Boecks occupied the professorial chair at Christiania (Oslo), separated in its tenure by Dr. Bidenkap, who had been Hutchinson's host and guide at Christiania. Just before his death, Caesar Boeck published the details of 24 cases of "benign miliary lupoids";[3] some cases involved the lungs, conjunctiva, bone, lymph nodes, spleen, and nasal mucosa, underlining the multisystemic nature of the disorder.

In all, three Professors Boeck of the same family were connected with Christiania University in the course of 90 years (1828–1917). All three were related to a Danish Captain of Artillery, Caesar Laesar Boeck (1766–1832) by one of his four marriages. The third Professor Boeck was another of Caesar's uncles, Christian Peter Bianco Boeck (1798–1877), who was Professor of Physiology, Comparative Anatomy, and Veterinary Medicine and one of the founders of the Norwegian Medical Society.

Fig. 2. Anomalous Disease of Skin of Fingers, &c. (Papillary psoriasis?).

Fig. 2 represents the hand of a man on which large, solid, livid patches of induration were present. These patches occurred, as is shown, on the middle finger, in the cleft between the middle and ring fingers and on the dorsum of the hand. They were abruptly margined, a good deal elevated and smooth. Their colour was almost purple. The artist has, I am sorry to say, not been very successful in representing the peculiarities described. There were patches of very similar character, but with less thickening, on the front of the left tibia. The patient was an elderly man, apparently in good health, but who had suffered much from gout. The patches had begun to appear two years before; they remained without alteration during the twelve months that he was under treatment, and I believe up to the time of his death, six years later. The following are the details.

John W—, æt. 58, was first under my care at the Hospital for Skin Diseases in January, 1869. He came on account of a number of peculiar patches of dark purplish colour on his extremities. The following description is taken from notes written at the time:—On the fronts of his legs, some of his fingers, and on one forearm, were a number of patches consisting in the first instance of distinct tubercles, which afterwards became confluent and then lost their tubercular character. The patches were peculiar chiefly on account of their dark purple colour; this tint seemed to depend partly upon venous congestion and partly upon deposit of colouring

CASE OF LIVID PAPILLARY PSORIASIS. 45

matter in the tissues, for although their margins could be made pale by pressure, no amount of squeezing altered the colour of the central parts. The patches were irregular in size and shape, distinctly raised above the general surface, their margins for the most part irregular and abruptly defined, and their surfaces smooth and almost glossy, or sometimes covered with thin dry epidermic scale. Their elevation above the surrounding skin was due in great part to œdema, for they could be made to pit by continued pressure, and in fact could be squeezed until almost all thickening disappeared. They were neither tender nor painful. The skin around them was slightly œdematous.

The patches were distributed on the whole symmetrically, but the symmetry was incomplete. There was a large patch on the front of each leg, that on the left being much the larger. Another large one was present on the back of each middle finger; on the right hand it involved nearly the whole finger, back and front, while in the left the patch occupied only the dorsum of the finger just above the knuckle. There were small separate tubercles of the same nature on the backs of the hands, but these were much more abundant on the right. On the left arm, there were two little patches, one above and the other below the elbow, whilst there were none at all on the right arm. Both hands were slightly swollen. The patient stated that the left leg was attacked first, and that the patch in that situation had been present for two years, while that on the right had existed only a couple of months. He was a stout florid man engaged at a coal-wharf and comfortably off. He was liable to attacks of gout, and considered that he had been subject to that disease for twenty-six years. From his account it seemed that he had had well-marked attacks, but that latterly they had been less severe. He was not aware that he inherited the gout. For years he had taken no beer at all, and only a little gin and water. In connection with the patches on the legs it should be stated that his veins were not markedly varicose.

He remained under care for very nearly twelve months,[1] and during that time the amount of swelling in connection with the patches diminished somewhat, but their colour remained the same. Some fresh patches appeared on the legs; a few of these were at the margins of the former ones, but others, separate ones, came at the backs of the calves, most of them being on the right, and only a single one on the left calf. He had an attack of gout in the metacarpo-phalangeal joint of his left forefinger while under treatment. No medicine had much effect on the eruption; he took at different times, colchicum and magnesia, arsenic, acid iron mixture, iodide of potassium, and simple alkaline mixture. No special local treatment was adopted, only an ointment of lead and mercury being ordered.

During a visit to Christiania in the summer of 1869, Dr. Bidenkap was kind enough to show me the collection of pathological drawings in the University Museum, and amongst these was one taken from a patient of Professor Boeck, showing a precisely similar condition of things to that delineated in my portrait. The only particulars that I could ascertain were that it was from the hand of a Swedish sailor, who appeared to be in good health, and who was not known to have suffered from gout. Professor Boeck told me that it was the only example of its kind that he had ever seen.

[1] I have learned whilst these pages have been passing through the press that this man has died within the last few weeks. From what his widow tells me, it is probable that the cause of death was bladder and kidney disease; I have not seen him for five years, and can therefore not add any further facts as to his skin malady. It is said to have persisted and to have extended. He had been under treatment for it at King's College Hospital, where his condition is said to have excited much interest.

Figure 1–2. Hutchinson's first published account of sarcoidosis, John W——.

Uncle Wilhelm enjoyed an international reputation based largely on a fallacy, for he believed that the soft sore was a mild and harmless form of syphilis. Bearing in mind the protective value of cowpox in preventing smallpox, he likewise advocated soft sore for the prevention of the late sequelae of syphilis. Nephew Caesar succeeded him in 1889 as head of the department of skin diseases at Christiania State Hospital. Caesar Boeck, age 44, was tall, charming, eloquent, and a splendid teacher; he returned both knowledgeable and mature after studying his subject abroad, notably in Vienna. He recognized the importance of throat infections as a cause of erythema nodosum, and he enjoyed describing a number of rare skin diseases. He inherited from his uncle the false belief that mercury was contraindicated in the early stages of syphilis. Between 1890 and 1910 nearly 2,000 syphilitics at the Rikshospital were admitted for in-patient placebo treatment lasting about four months. Caesar Boeck's successor, Professor Bruusgaard, followed up this series to define the natural history of untreated syphilis.

THE FRENCH SCHOOL

In 1889, Besnier described a patient with violaceous swellings of the nose, ears, and fingers, for which he coined the term *lupus pernio*.[4] He referred to Hutchinson's patient, John W——, but the distribution of the lesions was sufficiently dissimilar to justify his opinion that the two conditions were not identical. In 1892 Tenneson reported another example of lupus pernio and described the essential histology of "predominance of epithelioid cells and a variety of giant cells" in the skin lesions.[5]

MRS. MORTIMER

By 1898, Hutchinson had observed two other examples of lesions, and he, likewise, considered them to belong to the lupus family, for he recorded,[6]

I have to describe a form of skin disease which has, I believe, hitherto escaped especial recognition. It may not improbably be a tuberculous affection and one of the lupus family, but if so it differs widely from all other forms of lupus, both in its features and its course . . . The disease is characterised by the formation of multiple raised, dusky-red patches which have no tendency to inflame or ulcerate. They are very persistent, and extend but slowly. They occur in groups and are usually on both sides and almost symmetrical. The multiplicity of the patches, their occurrence in groups, their bilateral symmetry, and the absence of all tendency to ulcerate or form crusts, are features which separate the malady from lupus vulgaris. To none of the other forms of lupus has the malady any resemblance. The malady might perhaps be named Lupus Vulgaris Multiplex non-ulcerans, but for the present I prefer to recognise it, by the name of one of its subjects, as Mortimer's Malady.

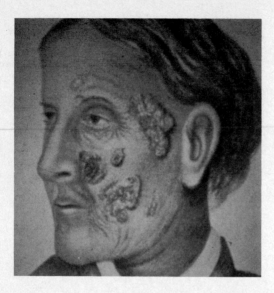

Figure 1–3. Mrs. Mortimer.

Mrs. Mortimer (Fig. 1–3) was 64 years old when she developed these lesions. Hutchinson presented her to a meeting of the Dermatological Society of London in 1895, at which time the consensus of opinion favoured the diagnosis of sarcoma, and urged skin biopsy for histological proof. Hutch-inson subsequently suggested this course of action to Mrs. Mortimer, with the result that he did not see her again for two years.

In 1897, Caesar Boeck presented to the Medical Society of Christiania (Oslo) a 34-year-old police constable with "multiple benign sarkoid of the skin" and drew attention to its similarity to Mortimer's malady.[7] Boeck's patient had developed several skin patches in the course of years and also had lymphadenopathy, particularly of the epitrochlear glands. Unlike Hutch-inson, Boeck was able to study the skin histologically and noted the sharply defined foci of epithelioid cells with some giant cells permeating the corium (Fig. 1–4; see also color plate 1). The lymph nodes were not examined. In his first communications, Boeck concluded that the condition may prove to be connected with the pseudo-leukaemias, but he subsequently amended this view in favour of a generalized disorder, allied in some way to tuberculosis.[8] Boeck's first patient died at the age of 80 with metastases from a hypernephroma, but at necropsy there was no remaining evidence of sarcoidosis. Interestingly, this patient was much earlier found to have a positive Kveim test.

MULTISYSTEM RECOGNITION

Further contributions drew attention to bone cysts, which Kienbock (1902) connected with syphilis[9] and Kreibich (1904) with lupus pernio[10] and

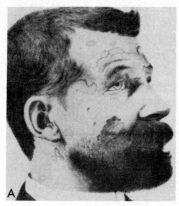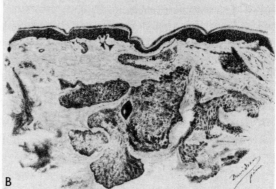

Figure 1–4. *A*, Boeck's patient was a police constable. The skin lesions resembled those of Mrs. Mortimer.

B, Boeck added the histology of epithelioid and giant cells.

which Jungling (1920) called *osteitis tuberculosa multiplex cystica*.[11] Darier and Roussy (1906) described subcutaneous nodules,[12] and Kuznitsky and Bittorf (1915), a dermatologist and a chest physician, respectively, drew attention to the pulmonary manifestations of sarcoidosis.[13] At this stage a pathological synthesis of the diverse aspects of the disease was due and was offered in an admirable Zambaco prize essay by Jorgen Schaumann (1936), who distinguished the condition from Hodgkin's malignant granuloma by calling it *lymphogranulome benign*.[14]

ERYTHEMA NODOSUM

The term *erythema nodosum* was introduced by Robert Willan in his work "On Cutaneous Diseases" published in parts between 1798 and 1808; among his fine coloured copperplate engravings is an illustration of erythema nodosum.[15] His classic description follows.

In erythema nodosum many of the red patches are large and rounded. The central parts of them are very gradually elevated and on the 6th or 7th day form hard and painful protruberances. From the 7th to the 10th, they constantly soften and subside without ulceration. On the 8th or 9th day, the red colour changes to bluish or livid, and the affected limb appears as if it had been severely bruised. This appearance remains for a week or ten days, when the cuticle begins to separate in scurf. The erythema nodosum usually affects the fore parts of the legs. I have only seen it in females, most of whom were servants. It is preceded by irregular shiverings, nausea, headaches and fretfulness with a quick unequal pulse and a whitish fur on the tongue. These symptoms continue for a week or more, but they usually abate on the appearance of the erythema.

He draws attention to the characteristic site, play of colours, and tenderness of the lesions; he refers to its predilection in females, and he underlines the constitutional upset that often precedes the rash. The description has not been bettered and is no less accurate today than it was in 1808. Physicians are still undecided about its pathogenesis, confused as to the relative frequency of its different causes, and have no better treatment than the Peruvian bark advocated by Willan.

LÖFGREN'S SYNDROME

The suggestion that erythema nodosum and bilateral hilar lymphadenopathy are frequent manifestations of sarcoidosis is more recent. Sven Löfgren (1946) of St. Goran's Hospital, Stockholm, analysed 185 cases of erythema nodosum and found 15 patients in whom sarcoidosis was probable despite lack of histological proof.[16] In a second Swedish survey published in 1953, he obtained histological proof of sarcoid tissue in one-fourth of a series of 113 patients with erythema nodosum and bilateral hilar lymphadenopathy.[17] In Great Britain, Kerley noted the radiological association,[18] and, eventually, histological proof of sarcoidosis was obtained by James, Thomson, and Willcox in a series of 27 patients with this syndrome.[19] From this series, it was not possible to define how often erythema nodosum was caused by sarcoidosis, but the association should particularly be sought in young adult women. From 1950 to 1959, 170 patients with erythema nodosum were personally studied and the frequency of sarcoidosis emphasized in this predominantly springtime phenomenon.[20]

OCULAR SARCOIDOSIS

The earliest descriptions of sarcoidosis drew attention to the cutaneous manifestations of the disease. Nearly 60 years were to elapse before it became accepted that the eye could be involved in a similar process. Jonathan Hutchinson was an able ophthalmologist as well as an observant dermatologist. He was, therefore, well qualified to note any possible association between inflammatory disease of the eye and the purple plaques he had described. His voluminous writings do not suggest that he had perceived such a link, although he does accurately record examples of subacute relapsing iridocyclitis with postcorneal precipitates, which may well have been due to sarcoidosis.[21]

Schumaker (1909) and Bering (1910) first drew attention to iritis accompanying sarcoidosis.[22, 23] In addition to lesions of the eye, they independently noted simultaneous involvement of the parotid and submaxillary glands. In view of positive tuberculin skin reactions, they concluded that their patients had tuberculous iritis.

HEERFORDT'S SYNDROME

The Danish ophthalmologist Heerfordt (1909) drew attention to *febris uveoparotidea subchronica*, characterized by uveitis and enlargement of the parotid glands.[24] The condition ran a chronic and usually febrile course, was frequently complicated by cranial nerve palsies, especially of the seventh cranial nerve, and was associated with pleocytosis of the cerebrospinal fluid. Heerfordt described three cases and referred to others in the literature. Since the latter had been ascribed to mumps, Heerfordt believed that his examples were due to the same cause.

During the following quarter century, the aetiology of Heerfordt's syndrome was fiercely debated. Two main schools of thought favoured either mumps or tuberculosis. Garland and Thompson (1933) favoured a tuberculous aetiology on the basis of their observations of one case and review of 46 examples from the literature.[25] They recommended that the syndrome be termed *uveoparotid tuberculosis*.

Controversy ended when Bruins-Slot (1936), Longcope and Pierson (1937), Pautrier (1937), and Waldenström (1937) identified uveoparotid fever as but another manifestation of sarcoidosis.[26-29] Jan Waldenström described five patients with uveoparotitis attending the medical, surgical, and ophthalmic clinics in Uppsala.[29] They had bilateral parotid gland enlargement and bilateral uveitis (see page 151). He produced compelling arguments identifying uveoparotitis as but another manifestation of sarcoidosis. His cogent reasons against the tuberculous aetiology were the negative tuberculin skin tests, the absence of caseation in the tissues, and the inability to isolate tubercule bacilli from the lesions. In favour of the identity of uveoparotitis and sarcoidosis, he cited the similarity of the skin lesions, the histology, and the occurrence in both of a similar hyperglobulinaemia.

BIOCHEMICAL ABNORMALITIES

In 1935, Salvesen described four patients in Oslo with sarcoidosis, three of whom had considerable hyperglobulinaemia of over 5 gm/100 ml.[30] The descriptive era had given way to the age of technology, and thereafter numerous reports indicated the biochemical derangement seen with sarcoidosis.[31]

KVEIM-SILTZBACH TEST

The other test that has added immeasurably to our knowledge of sarcoidosis is the Kveim-Siltzbach skin test reaction. Based on the hypothesis that sarcoidosis, like lymphogranuloma, might be a viral disease, Williams and Nickerson (1935) employed a skin test for its diagnosis.[32] Sarcoid tissue obtained from a skin lesion was suspended in saline, sterilized by heat, and inoculated intradermally into four patients with suspected sarcoidosis and four normal control subjects. Within 24 hours a firm red papule was observed in the first group and was still present a week later, whereas such a reaction was not observed in the control group. An Oslo dermatologist, Kveim (1941), added the important observation that these papules consisted of sarcoid tissue.[33] In one to four weeks following the intracutaneous inoculation of a heat-killed suspension of a sarcoid lymph node, he obtained histological evidence of sarcoid tissue from the injection site in 12 or 13 patients with sarcoidosis. Simultaneous control injections of Frei's antigen and tuberculin did not produce this response. Since this reaction did not occur in normal subjects, nor in patients with lupus vulgaris, he concluded that the papules were specific lesions due to an unknown agent and that the test served to differentiate sarcoidosis from tuberculosis. This simple, safe and specific out-patient technique has proved an important aid in the early diagnosis of sarcoidosis. Putkonen (1943) and Nelson (1949) emphasised its value as an index of activity of the disease.[34, 35] In a survey of the value of this test in 40 different countries, Siltzbach[36] showed that antigen prepared from the sarcoid spleen of one woman from New York has served as an effective test agent for detecting sarcoidosis throughout the world. This has also proved a convincing demonstration of the unitarian aetiology of the disease despite differences in sex and race and clinical, radiological, and immunological differences.

BIBLIOGRAPHY

It would be uncharitable to conclude any historical survey without drawing attention to the unique bibliography on sarcoidosis, spanning 1878 to 1963 initially and now constantly brought up to date by the United States National Library of Medicine. This was initiated by a group of devotees whose enthusiasm was kept burning brightly by Martin M. Cummings, Director of the National Library of Medicine, who has himself contributed authoritatively to the riddle of sarcoidosis.[37] This has been followed by a Japanese bibliography.[38]

WORLD CONFERENCES (Table 1–2)

First Conference (1958)

The Olympic torch was lit and the first conference was held from June 30 to July 2, 1958, in London. Until that time the clinicians had read each other's articles but did not know one another. They met in a spirit of

Table 1–2. International Conferences on Sarcoidosis

Year	City	Organiser	Delegates (No.)	Countries Represented (No.)	Communications (No.)
1958	London	D. Geraint James	22	8	22
1960	Washington	Martin Cummings	45	10	30
1963	Stockholm	Sven Löfgren	150	26	98
1966	Paris	Jude Turiaf	275	33	109
1969	Prague	Ladislav Levinsky	300	37	127
1972	Tokyo	Yutaka Hosoda	300	22	115
1975	New York	Louis Siltzbach	355	33	80
1978	Cardiff	W. Jones Williams	301	33	114
1981	Paris	Jacques Chretien	406	34	103*
1984	Baltimore	Carol Johns	307	29	92†

*84 posters.
†173 posters.

cordiality and camaraderie, and this spirit has pervaded all subsequent conferences (Fig. 1–5).

Second Conference[39] (1960)

This was arranged by the U.S. National Academy of Sciences–U.S. National Research Council in Washington D.C. from June 1 to 3, 1960, and masterminded by Dr. Martin Cummings. It was really a model for all

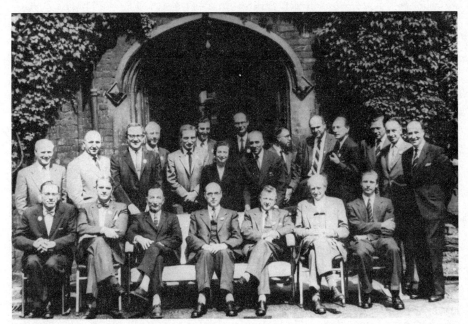

Figure 1–5. There were only 22 participants at the 1958 London Conference, including one woman, Dr. Ingrid Gilg.

conferences—intimate (we were just 45 active participants), academic, comfortable, genial, and fruitful (out of it came a working definition and exemplary proceedings).

Third Conference[40] (1963)

Even the weather smiled for Sven Löfgren, who was an outstanding organiser of the Stockholm meeting held from September 11 to 14, 1963, under the auspices of the International Union Against Tuberculosis. The representatives of 26 countries are listed in the excellent proceedings, edited by Sven Löfgren with the able assistance of Hans Bauer and Barbro Weist (Fig. 1–6).

Fourth Conference[41] (1966)

The Paris conference was held from September 12 to 15, 1966, under the genial presidency of Professor Jude Turiaf (Fig. 1–7) and was attended by 275 participants. The proceedings are a voluminous information–crammed 782 pages.

Fifth Conference[42] (1969)

The Prague Conference was held from June 16 to 21, 1'   nder the presidency of Professor Ladislav Levinsky and was attended t   delegates

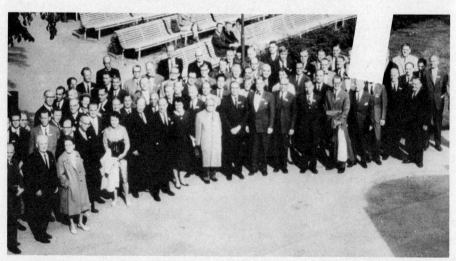

Figure 1–6. Large international participation in the Stockholm Conference (1963).

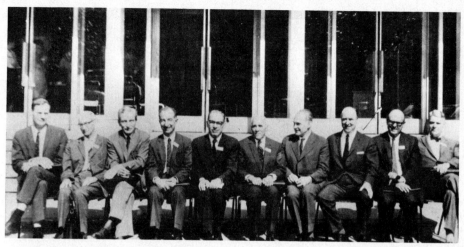

Figure 1–7. The International Committee on Sarcoidosis, assembled for the Paris Conference in 1966. From left to right: T.H. Hurley (Melbourne), E.A. Uehlinger (Zurich), J.S. Chapman (Dallas), H. Israel (Philadelphia), L.E. Siltzbach (New York), J. Turiaf (Paris), L. Levinsky (Prague), D. Geraint James (London), M.M. Cummings (Washington, D.C.), and S. Lofgren (Stockholm).

from 37 countries. It was also the XIVth Scientific Conference of the Medical Faculty of Charles University, so the August inaugural ceremony took place in the venerable Carolinum, beflagged with emblems of the state and this lovely old University (Fig. 1–8). It was in the Aula Magna, the assembly hall of Charles University since the 14th century, that Purkyne (1787–1869) made the historical first pronouncement that animal cells contained a nucleus. In

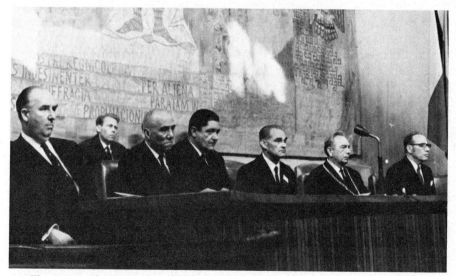

Figure 1–8. The inaugural ceremony at the Prague Conference (1969) in the venerable Aula Magna, the 14th century assembly hall of Charles University.

1969, the one-hundredth anniversary of the death of this Czech founder of modern physiology, histology, and of microscopy was commemorated. His motto was "Knowledge is Power," and this is also a good way of describing Levinsky's 653-page transactions of this conference.

Sixth Conference[43] (1972)

The Tokyo Conference was large and flamboyant and the only one to produce a special postage stamp. It is dated 72.9.15 for September 15, 1972, and next to the date can be seen VI ICS. This congress was well organised by Yutaka Hosoda and was held in Tokyo, with a post-congress meeting on treatment held in Kyoto.

Seventh Conference[44] (1975)

The seventh conference, held from October 6 to 10, 1975, in New York City under the presidency of Louis Siltzbach, introduced the most advanced immunological techniques not only for sarcoidosis but for other granulomatous disorders. The proceedings from this conference is a 751-page monograph containing 83 articles on all aspects—immunology, animal models and virology, physiology, epidemiology, diagnostic tests, treatment, and other granulomatous disorders.

Eighth Conference[45] (1978)

This was held from September 11 to 15, 1978, in Cardiff, the capital of Wales. It was organised by W. Jones Williams, who was ably assisted by B. H. Davies. This conference gave a fresh Celtic insight to sarcoidosis and other granulomatous disorders and was an important pioneer symposium on angiotensin-converting enzyme. Poster sessions were introduced successfully and will undoubtedly continue in future conferences.

The Transactions is a rich treasury of the latest information gleaned from 300 doctors contributing 114 communications. The epithelioid cell is scrutinised in detail, including electron microscopy and ion microprobe mass microanalysis. Its morphology is complemented by assessment of its active metabolism, and several exciting new secretory products, including angiotensin-secreting enzyme, are assessed and assigned a role for the first time. The newly recognised importance of bronchopulmonary alveolar macrophages is highlighted, immunological inhibitors are reviewed in detail, and the significance of such background factors as HLA antigens are analysed in relation to different ethnic groups.

Ninth Conference[46] (1981)

We returned to Paris from August 31 to September 4, 1981, under the leadership of Jacques Chretien (Fig. 1–9). For the first time, the immunology of sarcoidosis was tinged with monoclonal antibodies.

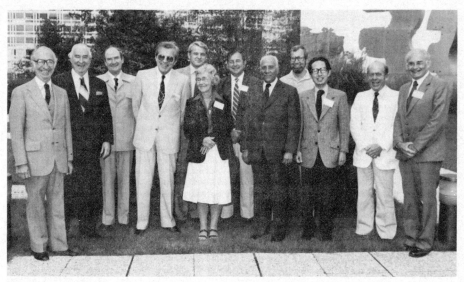

Figure 1–9. The International Committee on Sarcoidosis at the 1981 Paris Congress. From left to right: H. Israel, D. Geraint James (Executive Secretary), A. Douglas, J. Chretien (President), A. Hanngren, F. Basset, A. Teirstein, J. Turiaf, O. Selroos, Y. Hosoda, W. Jones Williams, L. Levinsky.

Tenth Conference (1984)

This was held on September 17 to 21, 1984, at the Johns Hopkins University Medical School, Baltimore, under the presidency of Dr. Carol Johns.

REFERENCES

1. Hutchinson J. Case of livid papillary psoriasis. *In* Illustrations of Clinical Surgery. London, J and A Churchill Ltd. 1:42, 1877.
2. Hutchinson J. On eruptions which occur in connection with gout. Arch Surg. 9:315, 1898.
3. Boeck C. Nochmals zur Klinik und zur stellung des "Benignen Miliarlupoids." Arch Derm Syph (Wein). 121:707, 1916.
4. Besnier E. Lupus pernio de la face. Ann Derm Syph (Paris). 10:333, 1889.
5. Tenneson M. Lupus pernio. Ann Derm Syph (Paris). 3:1142, 1892.
6. Hutchinson J. Case of Mortimer's malady. Arch Surg. 9:307, 315, 1898.
7. Boeck C. Multiple benign sarkoid of the skin. J Cutan Genitourin Dis. 17:543, 1899.
8. Boeck C. Fontgesetze, unter suchungen uber das multiple benigne sarkoid. Arch Derm Syph (Berlin). 73:301, 1905.
9. Kienbock R. Zur radiographischen anatomie und klinik der syphilitischen knockenerkankungen an extremitäten. Z Heilk (Chirug). 23:130, 1902.
10. Kreibich K. Uber lupus pernio. Arch Derm Syph (Wein). 71:3, 1904.
11. Jungling O. Ostitis tuberculosa multiplex cystica. Forschr Rontgesnstr. 27:375, 1920.
12. Darier J, Roussy G. Des sarcoides sous-cutaneous. Arch Med Exp. 18:1, 1906.
13. Kuznitsky E, Bittorf A. Boecksches sarkoid mit beteiligung innerer organe. Munch Med Wschr. 62:1349, 1915.

14. Schaumann J. Lupus pernio. Zambaco Prize Essay. Stockholm, PA Norstedt and Soner, 1934.
15. Willan R. On Cutaneous Diseases. London, J Johnson. 1:483, 1808.
16. Löfgren S. Erythema nodosum, studies on aetiology and pathogenesis in 185 adult cases. Acta Med Scand. 124 (Suppl):174, 1946.
17. Löfgren S. Primary pulmonary sarcoidosis. Acta Med Scand. 145:424, 1953.
18. Kerley P. The significance of the radiological manifestations of erythema nodosum. Br J Radiol. 15:155, 1942.
19. James DG, Thomson AD, Willcox A. Erythema nodosum as a manifestation of sarcoidosis. Lancet ii:218, 1956.
20. James DC. Erythema nodosum. Br Med J. 2:853, 1961.
21. Hutchinson J. Mabey's malady and lupus pernio. Arch Surg. 11:205, 1900.
22. Schumaker H. Tridocyclitis chronica. Munch Med Wschr. 56:2664, 1909.
23. Bering E. Zur kentnis des Boeckschen Sarkoids. Derm Z. 17:404, 1910.
24. Heerfordt CF. Uber eine "Febris uveo-parotidea subchronica" an der glandula parotis und der uvea des anges lokalisiert und haufig mit paresen crebrospinaler nerven kompliaiert. V Graefes Arch Ophthal. 70:254, 1909.
25. Garland HG, Thompson JG. Uveo-parotid tuberculosis (Febris uveoparotidea of Heerfordt). Quart J Med. 26:157, 1933.
26. Bruins-Slot W J. Ziekte von Besnier-Boeck en febris uveoparotidea (Heerfordt). Ned Tijdschr Geneesk. 80:2859, 1936.
27. Longcope WT, Pierson JW. Boeck's sarcoidosis. Bull Johns Hopkins Hosp 60:223, 1937.
28. Pautrier LM. Syndrome de Heerfordt et maladie de Besnier-Boeck Schaumann. Bull Soc Med Hop (Paris). 53:1608, 1937.
29. Waldenström J. Some observations on uveoparotitis and allied conditions with special reference to symptoms from nervous system. Acta Med Scand. 91:53, 1937.
30. Salvesen HA. The sarcoid of Boeck, a disease of importance in internal medicine; a report of four cases. Acta Med Scand. 86:127, 1935.
31. Studdy PR, Bird R, Neville E, James D G. Biochemical findings in sarcoidosis. J Clin Pathol. 33:528, 1980.
32. Williams RH, Nickerson DA. Skin reactions in sarcoid. Proc Soc Exp Biol (NY). 33:403, 1935.
33. Kveim A. En ny og spesifikk kirtan reaksjon ved Boecks sarcoid. Nord Med. 9:169, 1941.
34. Putkonen T. Uber die Kveim raction bei lymphogranulomatosis benigna. Acta Derm-Venereol (Stockh). 23:Suppl X, 1943.
35. Nelson CT. Kveim reaction in sarcoidosis. Arch Derm Syph (NY). 60:377, 1948.
36. Siltzbach LE. The Kveim test in sarcoidosis; a study of 750 patients. J Am Med Assoc. 178:476, 1961.
37. Mandel W, Thomas JH, Carman CT, McGovern JP. Bibliography on sarcoidosis 1878–1963. US Pub Health Publ 1213, Bibliography Series No. 51, 1964.
38. Ito Y. Bibliography on sarcoidosis. World Ed Pub Co Ltd, Tokyo, 1981.
39. Proceedings of the International Conference on Sarcoidosis. Am Rev Resp Dis. 84:171, 1961.
40. Proceedings 3rd International Conference on Sarcoidosis. Löfgren S (ed). Acta Med Scand Suppl 425, pp 309, 1964.
41. La Sarkoidose. Report of the 4th International Conference on Sarcoidosis. Turiaf J, Chabot J, James DG, Zatouroff M A (eds). Masson et Cie, Paris, pp 782, 1967.
42. Proceedings 5th International Conference on Sarcoidosis. Levinsky L, Macholda F (eds). Univ Karlova, Prague. pp 655, 1971.
43. Proceedings 6th International Conference on Sarcoidosis. Iwai K, Hosoda Y (eds). Univ Tokyo Press, Toyko. pp 666, 1974.
44. Proceedings 7th International Conference on Sarcoidosis and Other Granulomatous Diseases. Siltzbach LE (ed). NY Acad Sci. 278:751, 1976.
45. Sarcoidosis. Proceedings 8th International Conference on Sarcoidosis and Other Granulomatous diseases. Jones Williams W, Davies B H (eds). Alpha Omega Press, Cardiff. pp 774, 1980.
46. Proceedings 9th International Conference on Sarcoidosis and Other Granulomatous Diseases. Chretien J, Marsac J, Saltiel (eds). Pergamon Press, Paris. pp 676, 1983.

2

Descriptive Definition and Classification of Granulomatous Disorders

DESCRIPTIVE DEFINITION

Sarcoidosis is a multisystem disorder of unknown aetiology most commonly affecting young adults and presenting most frequently with bilateral hilar lymphadenopathy, pulmonary infiltration, and ocular and skin lesions. The diagnosis is established most securely when well-recognized clinicoradiographical findings are supported by histological evidence of widespread epithelioid cell granulomas in more than one system. Markers of activity of the disease include a positive Kveim-Siltzbach skin test, elevated serum angiotensin-converting enzyme (SACE) levels, hypercalciuria, hypercalcaemia, and intrathoracic uptake of radioactive gallium.

T4 helper cells are mobilized to all points of activity, where they cooperate with macrophages, leading to B cell overactivity. Activated T4 helper cells secrete a 20,000 dalton glycoprotein, interleukin 2, which leads to a tenfold clonal proliferation of the same T4 cells to augment their presence at sites of activity. This phenomenon does not include blood T lymphocytes; hence the relative anergy away from sites of activity.

The course and prognosis of the disorder correlate with the mode of onset; an acute onset usually heralds a self-limiting course with spontaneous resolution, whereas an insidious onset may be followed by relentless progressive fibrosis (Table 2–1).

Corticosteroids relieve symptoms, suppress granuloma formation, including those found by the Kveim-Siltzbach skin test, and normalise raised SACE levels.

CLASSIFICATION OF GRANULOMATOUS DISORDERS

The sarcoid granuloma is a non-specific response to many different antigens or irritants, some of which are recognised and others of which are still unknown. The inciting agents are persistent or poorly degradable. The

Table 2–1. Features Differentiating Acute Sarcoidosis from Chronic Sarcoidosis

Feature	Acute (Transient)	Chronic (Persistent)
Age (years)	< 30	> 40
Onset	Abrupt	Insidious
Chest x-ray	Bilateral hilar lymphadenopathy	Pulmonary infiltration/fibrosis
Eyes	Acute iritis, conjunctivitis, conjunctival nodules	Keratoconjunctivitis, chronic uveitis, glaucoma, cataracts
Skin	Erythema nodosum, vesicles, maculo-papular rash	Lupus pernio, plaques, scars, keloids
Parotitis Lymphadenopathy Splenomegaly Bell's palsy	Usually transient	Rarely permanent
Bone cysts	No	Yes
Histology	Epithelioid cell granulomas Alveolitis	Hyalinised granulomas Interstitial fibrosis
Acid phosphatase Leucine aminopeptidase	Increased	Normal
Calcium metabolism	Hypercalcaemia, hypercalciuria	Nephrocalcinosis
Urinary hydroxyproline	Increased	Normal
Kveim-Siltzbach test	Positive	May be negative
Tuberculin test	Negative	May become positive
K and NK cell	High	Unchanged
Gallium 67 uptake	High	Low
Angiotensin-converting enzyme	High	May be raised
Serum lysozyme	Increased	May be increased
Protein L1	Increased	Normal
Beta$_2$ microglobulin	High	May be raised
Circulating immune complexes process	Frequent	Less frequent
T helper:suppressor ratio in:	Lungs 10.5:1 Blood 0.8:1	1.4:1 1:1
Ia + T cells	Increased	Normal
Radioactive imipramine or propranolol reveal lung cell mass	Increased	Normal
Free light chains of immunoglobulins	Normal	Elevated
Lactoferrin	Increased	Normal
Serum collagenase	Elevated	Normal
Spontaneous remission	Frequent	Rare
Steroid therapy	Abortive effect	Symptomatic relief
Alternative drugs	Indomethacin	Chloroquine: Potaba methotrexate
Recurrence after steroid therapy	Rare	Frequent
Prognosis	Good	Poor

best-recognised causes are infections, chemicals, an enzyme defect, neoplasia, extrinsic allergic alveolitis, several immunological aberrations, and a miscellaneous group that cannot yet be classified (Table 2–2). Sarcoidosis is but one member of this large family of disorders, the basic denominator of which is a granulomatous process. This classification also provides the differential diagnosis and underlines the fact that sarcoidosis has numerous mimics.

Table 2–2. A Classification of Granulomatous Disorders

Infections

Bacteria	Brucella Francisella Proprioni Yersinia	*Spirochaetes*	Treponema pallidum T. carateum T. pertenue
Mycobacteria	M. tuberculosis M. kansasii M. avium M. leprae M. marinum BCG vaccine	*Protozoa* *Metazoa*	Toxoplasma Leishmania Toxocara Schistosoma
Fungi	Histoplasma Blastomyces Aspergillus Coccidioides Sporothrix Cryptococcus	*Viruses and Others*	Cat scratch disease Lymphogranuloma

Extrinsic Allergic Alveolitis	Farmer's lung Mushroom worker's lung Bagassosis Paprika splitter's lung	Bird fancier's lung Suberosis (cork dust) Maple bark stripper's lung Coffee bean lung
Chemicals	Beryllium Zirconium	Silica Starch
Neoplasia	Carcinoma Pinealoma Seminoma	Reticulosis Dysgerminoma Malignant nasal granuloma
Leucocyte oxidase defect	Chronic granulomatous disease of childhood	
Idiopathic	Sarcoidosis	

Crohn's disease	Giant cell arteritis
Primary biliary cirrhosis	Polyarteritis
Granulomatous hepatitis	Systemic lupus erythematosus
Whipple's disease	Hypogammaglobulinemia
Wegener's granulomatosis	Histiocytosis-X
Lymphatoid granulomatosis	Melkersson-Rosenthal syndrome
Churg-Strauss allergic granulomatosis	Peyronie's disease
Necrotising sarcoidal granulomatosis	Agammaglobulinaemia

Miscellaneous	Dermoid Sebaceous cyst Chalazion	Panniculitis Sea urchin spine injury Radiotherapy

The diagnosis of the various disorders of this family is most reliably made based on a combination of clinical and pathological evidence (see Chapter 15 for differential diagnosis). It is important to distinguish the multisystem disorder sarcoidosis from a non-specific local sarcoid-tissue reaction limited to one organ or system (Table 2–3).

Table 2–3. Differences Between the Multisystem Disorder Sarcoidosis and A Non-Specific Local Sarcoid-Tissue Reaction

Features	Sarcoidosis	Local Sarcoid-Tissue Reaction
Number of systems involved	Several	Usually one
Age group	20–50 years	Any
Chest radiograph	Abnormal in 88%	Normal
Slit lamp examination of eyes	Abnormal in 15%	Normal
Tuberculin test	Negative in 66%	Variable
Kveim-Siltzbach test	Positive in 75%	Negative
Elevated serum angiotensin-converting enzyme	In 60%	In 10%
Calcium metabolism	Abnormal in 20%	Normal
Response to steroids	Good	Variable
Other treatments	Phenylbutazone Chloroquine p-aminobenzoate Indomethacin Methotrexate	Depends on cause Anti-infective Immunosuppressive
Diet	Low calcium	Depends on cause

3

Pathology

INTRODUCTION

The central histological feature is non-caseating epithelioid cell granulomas in all tissues (Fig. 3–1). In recent years, emphasis has shifted away from the static morphology of the sarcoid granuloma to its more vital metabolic activity (Fig. 3–2). Instead of counting the inclusion bodies, an attempt is being made to quantitate its secretory products. The enzymes secreted by the granuloma include angiotensin-converting enzyme, lysozyme, glucuronidase, collagenase, and calcitriol. The serum angiotensin-converting enzyme activity has been harnessed into clinical use and has proved helpful in monitoring the activity of sarcoidosis (see Chapter 12).

THE SARCOID GRANULOMA

The granulomas consist of focal, tightly packed, interdigitating collections of modified macrophages and epithelioid cells, which often fuse to form multinucleate Langhans'-type giant cells and closely admixed lymphocytes. Central necrosis is usually absent but occasionally present in small amounts. As the lesions age they are infiltrated by fibroblasts with deposition of reticulin and hyalinised collagen (Fig. 3–3). Cellular inclusions, chiefly Schaumann's and asteroid bodies, are frequent and increase in number with aging.

EPITHELIOID CELL

These are certainly not modified epithelial cells, which give it the name, but are of bone marrow monocytic origin and thus by definition are modified macrophages.[1] They are distinguished from ordinary macrophages by their high content of synthesising enzymes,[2,3] prominent Golgi's complexes and muco-protein–containing secretory vesicles (Fig. 3–4), paucity of phagocytosis, and variable amounts of rough endoplasmic reticulum (RER).[4] Mature granulomas consist mainly of secretory cells (Type B), whereas developing granulomas are predominantly RER-rich cells (Type A) (Fig. 3–5; see also

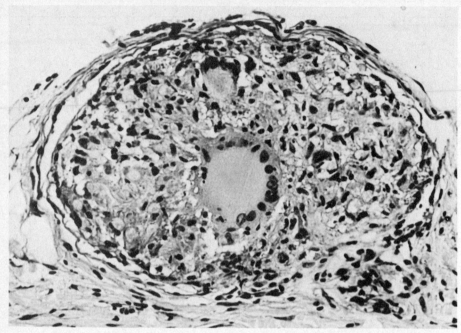

Figure 3–1. Sarcoid granuloma, epithelioid cells, Langhans-type giant cells, and admixed lymphocytes. H & E × 200.

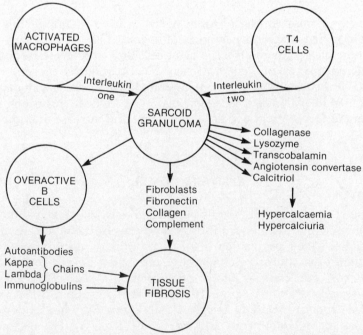

Figure 3–2. Sarcoid granuloma formation is an active metabolic process.

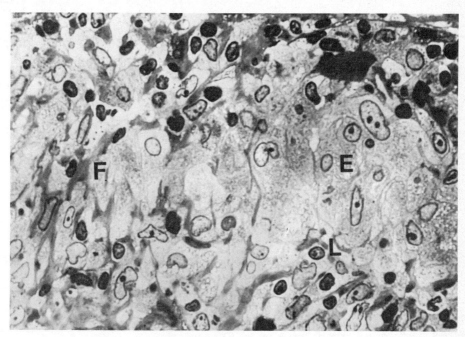

Figure 3–3. Sarcoid granulomas. E = Epithelioid cells; L = lymphocyte; F = developing fibrosis. Toluidine blue 1μ section × 1,200.

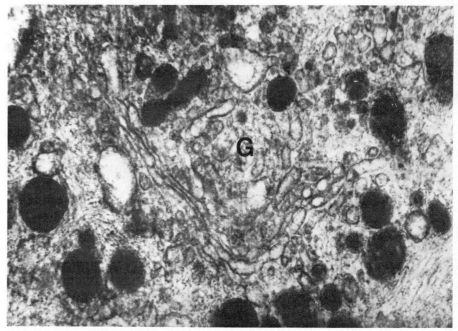

Figure 3–4. Epithelioid cell with Golgi's complexes (G) and secretory vesicles. Uranyl acetate and lead citrate × 15,000.

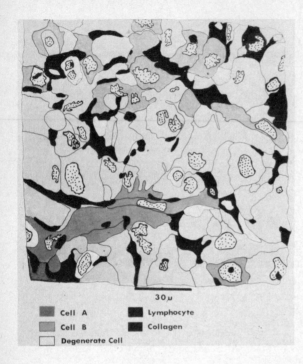

Figure 3–5. Electron micro-scope montage showing distri-bution of epithelioid cell types.

30 μ

■ Cell A   ■ Lymphocyte
■ Cell B   ■ Collagen
□ Degenerate Cell

color plate 2). Disaggregated epithelioid cells from experimental granulomas are less glass adherent, have fewer C3 receptors, and are less phagocytic than macrophages, and the transition from Type A to Type B cells is seen to occur with aging.[5] Broncho-alveolar lavage studies suggest that T helper cells accumulate at the site of maximal involvement and correlate with active disease,[6] and specific monoclonal antibody studies on tissue sections have shown that T helper cells predominate over T suppressor cells within the granulomas.[7]

INCLUSION BODIES

Schaumann's bodies (Fig. 3–6) consist of concentric laminated aggregated spherules, conchoidal bodies, made up of calcium/iron-impregnated lipo-mucoglycoproteins with central birefringent, possibly calcite, crystals.[8] They are densely basophilic and when fully formed look like a mulberry or raspberry. They form within epithelioid and giant cells and later become extracellular and invoke a foreign body–giant cell reaction. They are probably the end result of autophagocytic activity, are a form of "residual" body, and are not considered to contain any causative agent. Although common in sarcoidosis (88 per cent), they are not diagnostic, as they also occur in chronic beryllium disease (62 per cent), occasionally in Crohn's disease (10 per cent), rarely in tuberculosis (6 per cent), and very rarely in farmer's

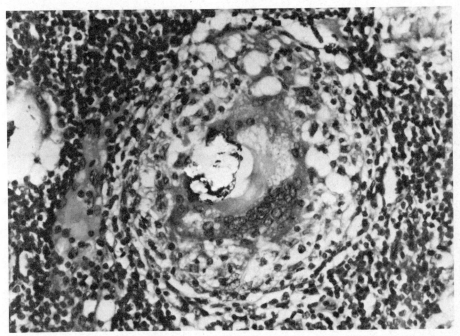

Figure 3–6. Schaumann's body within foreign body giant cell. H & E, polarised light × 200.

lung.[9] Hamazaki-Wesenburg bodies, consisting of intracellular yellow/brown granules, are also found in epithelioid/macrophages in a variety of diseases.[10] It is likely that these are also "residual" bodies related to Schaumann's bodies and likewise unrelated to any causative agent.[9] Asteroid, star-shaped bodies (Fig. 3–7) commonly occur within giant cells but again are present in many other granulomatous diseases. Known to be lipoprotein, they are now regarded as part of the cytoskeleton and consist of microfilaments and microtubules.[11]

LYMPHOKINES

What is the relation between the form and function of the cells in the epithelioid granulomas? There is increasing evidence that, although epithelioid cells are of mononuclear and hence phagocytic origin, they are primarily synthesising cells. A number of products have been suggested, in particular lymphokine-like substances[12] and angiotensin-converting enzyme.[13]

Lymphokines, defined as products of antigen-stimulated sensitised T lymphocytes, play an important role in the formation of epithelioid cell granulomas. They affect macrophages in a number of ways, inhibit migration and spreading, increase adhesion and aggregation, and activate a variety of intracellular enzymes; these may contribute to the classical tightly packed

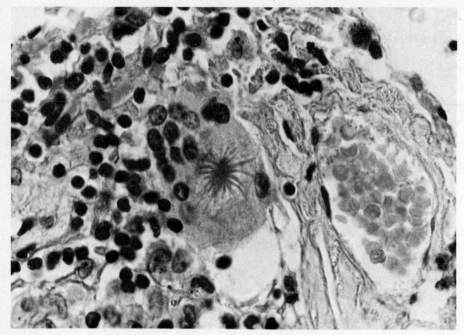

Figure 3–7. Asteroid body in giant cell. H & E × 400.

"knot" of cells constituting the granuloma. The process would be considerably enhanced by the additional secretion of lymphokine-like substances from epithelioid cells.

PROGRESSION TO FIBROSIS

With aging, the granulomas are infiltrated by fibroblasts, and early fibrosis is recognised by increasing deposition of intracellular reticulin (Fig. 3–8), which is gradually replaced by formed banded collagen (Fig. 3–9). Later the collagen is frequently transformed into structureless eosinophilic hyaline material (Fig. 3–10). Collagen is not just inert scar tissue but exists in many different forms. It is likely that some forms are completely reversible (Type III) and that progression to end-stage scar tissue is dependent on the balance of the various types. Knowledge of the exact composition of hyaline is urgently required. Not all van Gieson's-positive collagen leads to permanent scar tissue; occasionally patients with lung biopsies with granulomas and fibrosis make a complete clinical recovery with return to radiological and physiological normality.

Fibrosis is dependent upon a very complex cellular interaction (Fig. 3–11). The central factor is the continuing stimulus of a persistent causative agent ("antigen"), which is directly responsible for granuloma formation.

The "antigen" also activates thymic (T, Tm, and Tg) and bursal (B) lymphocytes. T lymphocyte–produced lymphokines are capable of attracting and activating circulating monocytes, macrophages, and probably epithelioid cells. B lymphocytes, activated directly or indirectly by T cell subsets, produce a variety of immunoglobulins, which contribute to the formation of immune complexes. It is possible that altered collagen and fibronectin may contribute to immune complex formation. Macrophages are known to produce a variety of factors that can influence fibrosis, including fibronectin (recruitment factor) and growth factor (replication), which influence fibroblasts to produce collagen I fibrosis. This is inhibited by colchicine and prostaglandin E2, augmented by interleukin 1, and uninfluenced by steroids.

The relation of activated macrophages to the development of fibrosis is well illustrated by various types of pneumoconiosis. Coal is a relatively inert dust that fills the macrophages but causes virtually no activation, so the dust foci of simple coalworker's pneumoconiosis shows little or no fibrosis. Fibrotic nodules occur with increasing silica content of coal. Silica stimulates macrophage recruitment, resulting in the formation of dense whorled fibrotic nodules. The immune complexes of rheumatoid arthritis may likewise stimulate activated macrophages to form Caplan nodules of fibrosis,[14] and tubercle bacilli may contribute to progressive massive fibrosis.[15]

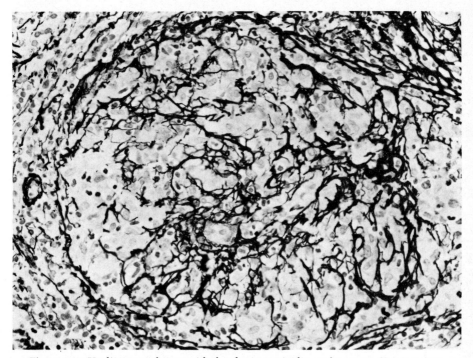

Figure 3–8. Healing granulomas with developing reticulin replacement. H & E × 350.

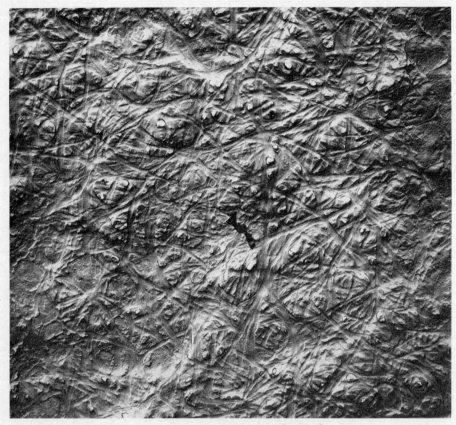

Figure 3–9. Collagen replacement of granulomas. Silver replication cast × 30,000.

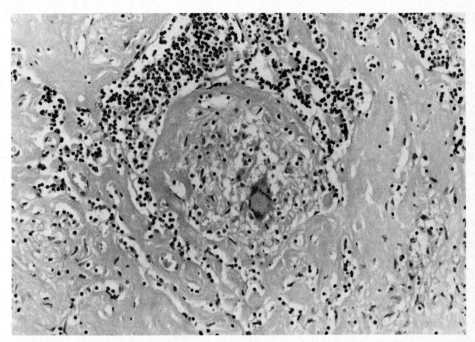

Figure 3–10. Granuloma remnant extensively replaced by hyalinised collagen. H & E × 120.

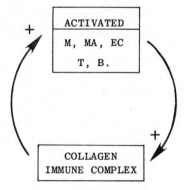

Figure 3–11. Secondary "antigen" in granuloma formation.

PRIMARY
'ANTIGEN'

+

ACTIVATED

M, MA, EC

T, B.

+

COLLAGEN
IMMUNE COMPLEX

(Secondary antigen)

M - Monocyte   EC - Epithelioid cells

MA - Macrophage   T - T lymphocytes

B - B lymphocytes

Table 3–1. Distribution of Histological Confirmation in a Series of 818 Patients with Sarcoidosis Compared with the Worldwide Survey

Tissue	Royal Northern Hospital		Worldwide	
	Number	%	Number	%
Lymph node	121	30	960	46
Skin	114	29	237	11
Liver	96	25	198	10
Miscellaneous	60	16	1395	33
Total	391	100	2062	100
Positive Kveim	550/657	84	1714/2189	78

DIAGNOSTIC HISTOLOGY

The diagnosis of sarcoidosis is only secure when consistent clinical and radiographic features are supported by histological proof of sarcoid tissue from at least one, and preferably more than one, system. Evidence of one without the other is insufficient, for clinical or radiological manifestations alone carry too wide a differential diagnosis. Likewise, histological evidence of sarcoid tissue alone is non-specific, for there are numerous causes of granuloma formation peculiar to each system and tissue (see Chapter 15).

Between 1950 and 1975, several popular methods of obtaining histological confirmation were used (Tables 3–1 and 3–2).[16]

Table 3–2. Number of Patients and Patterns of Histological Confirmation in A Worldwide Survey

Centre	Tissue					Total Histological Confirmation
	Bronchus	Lymph Node	Skin	Liver Biopsy	Other Tissues	
London	0	100	82	76	42	300
New York	0	89	31	12	33	155
Paris	243	49	16	12	44	364
Los Angeles	2	53	19	38	32	144
Tokyo	0	118	19	9	10	156
Reading	45	46	33	9	78	211
Lisbon	16	36	18	9	7	85
Edinburgh	0	109	16	10	29	164
Novi Sad	15	115	8	15	17	170
Naples	7	212	1	0	1	221
Geneva	1	33	4	19	24	81
Total Number	329	960	247	209	317	2062
Total %	14	47	12	10	17	100

Bronchoscopy (see Chapter 5)

The popularity of fibreoptic bronchoscopy has brought about many changes. The flexible forceps biopsy secures bronchial and lung tissue and also permits a harvest of cell-rich broncho-alveolar lavage fluid. Sarcoid tissue histology is obtained in about 80 per cent of patients by this technique. This suggests that Stage 3 pulmonary sarcoidosis is not just end-stage fibrosis but also indicates evidence of continuing activity.

Skin (see Chapter 7)

Original observations on sarcoidosis stemmed from dermatologists, and skin biopsy remains a simple and specific means for confirming the diagnosis. Beware of confusion due to local non-specific sarcoid granulomas from silica, talc, scars, meibomian cysts, and old ruptured sebaceous cysts.

Lymph Node Biopsy (see Chapter 9)

Lymph node biopsy has been universally favoured over the years as a quick means of confirming the diagnosis of sarcoidosis. Its popularity is evident in the world series (see Tables 3–1 and 3–2), for lymph node biopsy was positive in 960 (47 per cent) patients—as popular as all other techniques combined. Any accessible lymph node is convenient, but the right scalene lymph node is the most popular. The mediastinal lymph node chain ascends on the right side, and right paratracheal lymphadenopathy is very frequent, leading to the high incidence of positive right scalene node biopsies. Variations in the technique led to mediastinoscopy and mediastinotomy, but fibreoptic bronchoscopy has now overshadowed these techniques.

Liver Biopsy (see Chapter 11)

Hepatic granulomas noted by the pathologist in aspiration liver biopsy specimens fall into three groups:[17]
1. The cause is seen under the microscope. The granuloma surrounds ova of *Schistoma mansoni* or tubercle bacilli are found in a caseous granuloma.
2. The cause is not discernible, but circumstantial evidence points to the diagnosis. The granuloma is adjacent to damaged bile ducts in primary biliary cirrhosis. In Q fever there may be a distinctive pattern of epithelioid cells, segmented leukocytes, and fibrin surrounding fat vacuoles. Extensive caseous necrosis points to tuberculosis in this group. Clusters of fibrosing granulomas in portal tracts suggest sarcoidosis.

3. There are miscellaneous but largely unidentifiable causes obvious to the histologist alone. Identification demands close clinicopathological collaboration. This may bring to light drug hypersensitivity with tissue and peripheral blood eosinophilia. It is also possible to identify in this group the ill-defined immunological hepatic granulomas with constitutional features suggesting circulation of immune complexes.

The granuloma in sarcoidosis is large, well-organised, and usually near portal tracts. There may be multinucleate giant cells and other inclusions. Central necrosis is minimal, and the reticulin network is well preserved. A thin peripheral ring of lymphocytes surrounds the lesion; healing is by sclerosis. The granuloma is converted into an acellular mass of hyaline material. Since the hepatic lesions are focal and fibrosis is restricted to healing lesions, sarcoidosis does not produce the diffuse fibrosis and nodular regeneration seen in cirrhosis.[18, 19]

The Spleen (see Chapter 9)

Selroos has pioneered fine needle aspiration biopsy of the spleen.[20] The aspiration device consists of a 0.7- to 0.8-mm needle on a 10- to 20-ml disposable syringe with a Luer adaptor. The needle is inserted into the tenth intercostal space, 3 to 4 cm dorsal to the midaxillary line. Local anaesthesia is unnecessary. The patient holds his breath in mid expiration. The aspirated material is spread on glass slides, air dried, and stained with May-Grünwald-Giemsa stains. The only contraindications to the procedure are an overt haemorrhagic diathesis and a platelet count below 100,000/mm.[3] Selroos does this procedure even when the spleen is not enlarged; he has used this technique in over 600 patients and regards it as his first choice for obtaining diagnostic histology. It is a simple, safe bedside technique in his hands, and he stresses its advantage of providing histological confirmation of sarcoidosis within one hour.

Peritoneoscopy

Many gastroenterologists favour peritoneoscopy because it provides the advantage of visualising the viscera together with an easy means of obtaining histology. Tachibana has studied 65 sarcoidosis patients with asymptomatic hepatic lesions by peritoneoscopy and was able to obtain biopsies of liver granulomas in 51 of these patients by direct vision.[21] In 6 of these 51 patients he also noted nodules on the surface of the spleen. Biopsies of these splenic nodules revealed characteristic sarcoid granulomas.

This technique not only visualises the granulomatous nodules on the surface of the liver and spleen and allows direct vision biopsy, but Tachibana has also been able to take the most elegant colour photographs as a permanent record of these abnormalities.

Muscle Biopsy (see Chapter 10)

Muscle biopsy is regarded in very much the same way as aspiration liver biopsy. The small sarcoid granulomas submitted in the biopsy may only become evident on multiple serial sections. Muscle involvement occurs as frequently as involvement of any other tissues in both acute and chronic forms of the disorder. What is important for the future is that those who do muscle biopsies should endeavour to correlate myositis and other types of muscle involvement with the clinical picture elsewhere and to make sure that they are dealing with multisystem sarcoidosis and not a local sarcoid-tissue reaction in muscle. The biopsy is usually taken from gastrocnemius muscle and fixed in 10 per cent neutral formalin. Granulomas are found in about one-half of biopsy series, if serial sections are made.[22]

Minor Salivary Gland Biopsy

Biopsy of the minor salivary glands is a simple out-patient technique. The lower lip is everted and a chalazion clamp is applied at random. Local anaesthesia is injected into a mental foramen; an incision 4 to 6 mm long and 1 to 2 mm deep is made, and one or two minor salivary glands are excised. The incision is closed with silk or plain gut sutures. Non-caseating granulomas were obtained in 58 per cent of patients with sarcoidosis in one series of 75 patients.[23] Granulomas were obtained in one of three patients with a normal chest radiograph and in three-fifths of patients with hilar adenopathy or pulmonary involvement. The late Dr. Siltzbach was also an advocate of gum biopsy. It is a simple technique, and sarcoid granulomas are often found, particularly if the small specimen is subjected to serial biopsy. Their presence underlines the fact that sarcoid granulomas are widely disseminated.

Conjunctiva (see Chapter 6)

Blind biopsy of the normal conjunctiva is unrewarding. If it were fruitful, then ophthalmologists would not need to turn to other biopsies for confirmation of sarcoidosis.

Sarcoid tissue is obtained from obvious phlyctenules. Biopsy of the lacrimal glands is valuable in the small group of black patients with florid sarcoid lesions including enlarged lacrimals.

Having painted this gloomy British picture of the place of "blind" conjunctival biopsy in the assessment of sarcoidosis, we redress the balance by quoting the much rosier experience of Anni Karma (Finland),[24] who analysed a series of 79 patients with ocular sarcoidosis and obtained histological evidence of conjunctival granulomas in 37, an incidence of 17 per cent of 218 patients examined.

One pitfall cannot be over-emphasised, namely, that conjunctival biopsy may produce non-specific foreign body giant cell granulomas, and these must not be misconstrued as the granulomas of sarcoidosis (see Table 2–3).

Upper Respiratory Tract (see Chapter 5)

Our series of 818 patients with sarcoidosis includes 53 (6 per cent) patients with sarcoidosis of the upper respiratory tract (SURT). We obtained histological evidence of sarcoidosis from several sites, often from more than one site. These sites included nasal mucosa in 36 patients, laryngeal and pharyngeal mucosa in 8, sinuses in 8, and parotid gland involvement in 10 patients. When granulomas are found on biopsy of the upper respiratory tract, it is important to decide whether they represent multisystem sarcoidosis or whether they are due to tuberculosis, Wegener's granulomatosis, leprosy, or local reactions to foreign material.[25]

The Heart (see Chapter 10)

Myocardial sarcoidosis is difficult to recognize clinically. It does not pose a great problem if a patient with florid multisystem sarcoidosis develops bundle branch block, arrhythmias, congestive cardiac failure, pericarditis, or clinical evidence of cardiomyopathy. However, sudden death due to myocardial sarcoidosis may occur in an otherwise healthy asymptomatic individual. Between these two extremes lie patterns of involvement, including cardiomyopathy, when endocardial biopsy may be indicated. This technique is easily performed by those accustomed to cardiac catheterisation. It can be done at the same time as catheterisation of the left or right side of the heart. It is recommended by Japanese workers as an aid to the diagnosis of myocardial sarcoidosis, when serial changes show worsening of the ECG or vectorcardiography reveals disturbances of conduction.[26]

Kveim-Siltzbach Skin Test

Since those early days recounted in Chapter 1, there has been a generation of experience gained regarding the course and prognosis of sarcoidosis around the world with a retrospective comparison of large, intensively investigated series. The 11-city survey indicates that the Kveim test remains reliable and helpful in three different continents of the world. It was positive in 1,714 of 2,189 (78 per cent) patients tested with insignificant false-positive reactions (Table 3–3).

Kveim-Siltzbach antigen is a saline suspension of human sarcoid tissue prepared from the spleen of a patient suffering from active sarcoidosis.[27] The

Table 3–3. Results of Kveim-Siltzbach Skin Tests in 2,189 Patients with Sarcoidosis in 11 Cities

| | | Kveim-Siltzbach Skin Test | |
| | | Positive | |
Centre	Patients Tested	No.	%
London	466	384	82
New York	311	285	92
Paris	261	202	77
Los Angeles	50	36	72
Tokyo	141	76	54
Reading	408	331	81
Lisbon	55	43	78
Edinburgh	222	141	64
Novi Sad	205	167	81
Naples	27	15	56
Geneva	43	36	84
Overall	2,189	1,714	78

*Data from James DG et al. A worldwide review of sarcoidosis. Ann NY Acad Sci. 278:321, 1976.

antigen, 0.15 ml, is injected intradermally very superficially into the flexor surface of the forearm, and the inoculation site is observed for the development of a visible and palpable nodule during the ensuing six weeks. Any palpable nodule is biopsied, usually one month after the injection, using a Hayes-Martin drill. This core of tissue is serially sectioned for evidence of sarcoid tissue or a foreign body–giant cell reaction. This diagnosis is made blind; that is, without knowledge of the clinical picture. A Kveim-Siltzbach test is reported as positive if the intradermally injected antigen produces a nodule in the course of four weeks and this nodule shows evidence of sarcoid tissue, as distinct from a foreign body–giant cell reaction.

A parallel may be drawn between the Kveim-Siltzbach skin test and the beryllium patch test in beryllium disease, the zirconium skin reaction in patients with zirconium deodorant granulomas, and the lepromin reaction in leprosy. All tests are specific for their own disease states. That these disease states are a form of hypersensitivity phenomenon is suggested by several facts: (1) they occur in patients who have been in contact with, for example, beryllium or zirconium; (2) they are not positive before contact; (3) a positive result can be obtained using extremely high dilutions of the element; and (4) the reaction is specific.

Several factors influence the Kveim-Siltzbach reaction, which must still be regarded as a crude but most useful biological test. Potent antigen is essential, and this means that it must be obtained from the spleen of a patient with active sarcoidosis.[28] Another important factor is the histologist's interpretation of the biopsy material; an inexperienced observer could confuse sarcoid tissue with a non-specific foreign body–giant cell reaction, particularly if doubly refractile crystals are not sought by polarised light.[29]

Finally, the Kveim-Siltzbach test is suppressed by oral corticosteroids, just as any sarcoid tissue is suppressed by these potent anti-inflammatory agents. An occasional false-positive result is inevitable with a biological test of this kind, but a figure of less than 2 per cent is acceptable.

It is particularly helpful when histological confirmation is otherwise lacking or equivocal. It is useful in the differential diagnosis of diffuse pulmonary mottling, uveitis, and erythema nodosum and in distinguishing hepatic granulomas. It is also worth performing in obscure cases of subacute meningitis or cranial nerve palsies. It is negative in patients with non-specific local sarcoid-tissue reactions and in all other granulomatous disorders.

Attempts have also been made to develop *in vitro* Kveim tests.[30–32] These depend on the production of lymphokines, macrophage/polymorphonuclear migration inhibition, and transformation factors from Kveim-stimulated lymphocytes. The advantages of such tests include a rapid result in two days, no need for biopsy, and, therefore, avoidance of histological misinterpretation. Some Kveim suspensions have, however, provided an unacceptably high-positive rate in non-sarcoid patients,[29] so that this technique has not been widely accepted.

REFERENCES

1. Spector WG, Mariano M. Macrophage behaviour in experimental granulomas. *In* van Furth R (ed): Mononuclear Phagocytes in Immunity Infection & Pathology. Oxford, Blackwell. p 927, 1975.
2. Williams D, Jones Williams W, Williams JE. Enzyme histochemistry of epithelioid cells in sarcoidosis and sarcoid-like granulomas. J Clin Pathol 97:705, 1969.
3. Muller-Hermelink HK, Kamiyama R, Kaiserling E, Lennert K. Lymph node findings in sarcoidosis, light microscopical, ultrastructural and enzyme histochemical results. *In* Jones Williams W, Davies BH (eds): Sarcoidosis. Cardiff, Alpha Omega Press. p 23, 1980.
4. James EMV, Jones Williams W. Fine structure and histochemistry of epithelioid cells in sarcoidosis. Thorax. 29:115, 1974.
5. Williams GT. Isolated epithelioid cells from disaggregated BCG granulomas—some functional studies. J Pathol. 136:15, 1982.
6. Hunninghake GW, Crystal RG. Pulmonary sarcoidosis: a disorder mediated by excess helper T-lymphocyte activity in sites of disease activity. N Engl J Med. 8:429, 1981.
7. Semenzato G, Pezzuto A, Chisoli M, Pizzola G. Redistribution of T lymphocytes in the lymph nodes of patients with sarcoidosis. N Engl J Med. 306:48, 1982.
8. Jones Williams W. The Nature and origin of Schaumann bodies. J Path Bact. 69:193, 1960.
9. Jones William W, Williams D. The properties and development of conchoidal bodies in sarcoid and sarcoid-like granulomas. J Path Bact. 96:491, 1968.
10. Doyle WF, Brahman HD, Bergen JH. The nature of yellow brown bodies in peritoneal lymph nodes. Arch Pathol. 96:320, 1973.
11. Cain H, Kraus B. The ultrastructure and morphogenesis of asteroid bodies in sarcoidosis and other granulomas disorders. *In* Jones Williams W, Davies BH (eds): Sarcoidosis. Cardiff, Alpha Omega Press. p 30, 1980.
12. Jones Williams W. Sarcoidosis—1977. Beitr Path. 160:325, 1977.
13. Silverstein E, Friedland J, Pertschuk LP. Sarcoidosis pathogenesis. Mechanisms of angiotensin converting enzyme elevator, epithelioid cell localisation and induction of macrophages and monocytes in culture. *In* Jones Williams W, Davies BH (eds): Sarcoidosis. Cardiff, Alpha Omega Press. p 246, 1980.

14. Gough J, Rivers D, Seal RME. Pathological studies of modified pneumoconiosis in coal miners with rheumatoid arthritis (Caplan's syndrome). Thorax. 10:9, 1955.
15. Wagner JC. Aetiological factors in complicated coal workers' pneumoconiosis. Ann N Y Acad Sci. 200:401, 1972.
16. James DG, Neville E, Siltzbach LE, Turiaf J, Battesti JP, Sharma OP, et al. A worldwide review of sarcoidosis. Ann NY Acad Sci. 278:321, 1976.
17. Neville E, Piyasena KHG, James DG. Granulomas of the liver. Postgrad Med J. 51:361, 1975.
18. Klatskin G. Hepatic granulomata: problems in interpretation. Ann NY Acad Sci. 278:427, 1979.
19. MacSween RNM. In MacSween RNM, Anthony PP, Scheuer PJ (eds): Pathology of the Liver. Edinburgh, Churchill Livingstone. p 417, 1979.
20. Selroos O. Fine-needle aspiration biopsy of the spleen in diagnosis of sarcoidosis. Ann NY Acad Sci. 278:517, 1976.
21. Tachibana T. Peritoneoscopy of sarcoid hepatosplenomegaly. Ann NY Acad Sci. 278:520, 1976.
22. Stjernberg N, Cajander S, Truedsson H, Uddenfeldt P. Muscle involvement in sarcoidosis. Acta Med Scand. 209:213, 1981.
23. Nessan VJ, Jacoway JR. Biopsy of minor salivary glands in the diagnosis of sarcoidosis. New Engl J Med. 301:922, 1979.
24. Karma A. Ophthalmic changes in sarcoidosis. Acta Ophthal Suppl. 141, 1979.
25. Neville E, Mills RGS, James DG. Sarcoidosis of the upper respiratory tract and its relation to lupus pernio. Ann NY Acad Sci. 278:416, 1976.
26. Numao Y, Sekiguchi M, Fruie T, Matsui Y, Izumi T, Mikami R. A study of cardiac involvement in 963 cases of sarcoidosis by ECG and endomyocardial biopsy. In Jones Williams W, Davies BH (eds): Sarcoidosis. Cardiff, Alpha Omega Press, 1980, p. 607.
27. Chase MW. Preparation and standardisation of Kveim-testing antigen. Rev Resp Dis. 84:5, 1961.
28. Siltzbach LE. Qualities and behaviour of satisfactory Kveim suspensions. Ann NY Acad Sci. 278:665, 1976.
29. Jones Williams W, Seal RME, Davies KJ. International Kveim histology trial. Ann NY Acad Sci. 278:687, 1976.
30. Hardt F, Wanstrup J. Sarcoidosis, an 'in vitro' Kveim reaction based on the leukocyte migration test. Acta Path Microbiol Scand. 76:493, 1969.
31. Kalden JR, Becker FW, Kroll P, Deicher H. The 'in vitro' Kveim reaction in sarcoidosis and other diseases. An evaluation of the specificity of the test. In Iwai K, Hosada Y (eds): Proc VI Internat Conf Sarcoidosis. Tokyo Univ Press. p 39, 1974.
32. Jones Williams W, Pioli E, Jones DJ, Calcraft B, Johnson AJ, Dighero H. 'In vitro' Kveim induced macrophage inhibition factor, KMIF test, in sarcoidosis, Crohn's disease and tuberculosis. In Iwai K, Hosada Y (eds): Proc VI Internat Conf Sarcoidosis. Tokyo Univ Press. p 44, 1974.

4

Multisystem Clinical Features

MATERIAL

Our clinical data are based on the long-term and close follow-up of 818 patients attending a special Sarcoidosis Clinic in London held weekly during the last 30 years (1951 to 1981) (Table 4–1). We have personally examined, investigated, treated, and guided all these patients throughout their illness, irrespective of which system was involved. This provides homogeneity in the management of sarcoidosis in London.

Since this is a one-man view of sarcoidosis, we have added international breadth and heterogeneity by conducting a worldwide survey and comparing sarcoidosis in Britain and in other centres throughout the World (Table 4–2). The worldwide series comprises 3,676 patients attending 11 sarcoidosis clinics in 9 different countries. The data are surprisingly similar.

Since sarcoidosis is multisystemic, there were several patterns of presentation, but the majority were respiratory, ophthalmic, or dermatological (Table 4–3). General examination of the patient must be thorough (Fig. 4–1). It is incomplete unless accompanied by a chest radiograph, slit lamp examination of the eyes, and estimation of the 24-hour urine calcium level.

AGE, SEX, AND RACE (Tables 4–4 and 4–5)

Of the 818 patients in the Royal Northern Hospital series, 392 (48 per cent) presented under the age of 30 and 604 (74 per cent) under the age of 40. Among those under the age of 30, 254 (65 per cent) patients had an acute course, whereas 120 (31 per cent) were more chronic. There was a small majority of females in both the London and worldwide series. Nearly all the patients in the London series were born in the United Kingdom, but there was also a significant minority of migrants from Ireland and the West Indies (see Table 4–1). In the worldwide survey the ethnic background was that of the investigating country. The Tokyo series was entirely Japanese. The majority of patients in all centres were white (79 per cent overall), and only in New York and Los Angeles were there a majority of black patients.

Table 4–1. Features of Sarcoidosis in the Royal Northern Hospital Series Compared with a Worldwide Survey

Feature	Royal Northern Hospital		Worldwide	
	Number	*%*	*Number*	*%*
Female	500	61	2,082	57
Presentation under 40 years of age	604	74	2,504	68
Caucasian	728	89	—	—
West Indian	81	10	—	—
Intrathoracic	700	88	3,224	87
Ocular	224	27	—	—
Erythema nodosum	251	34	640	17
Lupus pernio	35	4	—	—
Other skin lesions	113	14	324	9
Ocular lesions	224	27	539	15
Parotid enlargement	52	6	160	4
Nervous system	77	9	134	4
Bone	31	3	109	3
Lymph nodes and spleen	326	39	1,031	28
Lymphadenopathy	225	27	—	—
Splenomegaly	101	12	—	—
Hepatomegaly	82	10	—	—
Heart	27	3	—	—
Lacrimal gland	22	3	—	—
Kidney	10	1	—	—
Upper respiratory tract	53	6	—	—
Systemic corticosteroid therapy	344	42	1,738	47
Mortality due to				
Sarcoidosis	25	3	84	2.2
Other causes	23	3	54	1.4
Skin tests				
Positive Kveim-Siltzbach	550/657	84	1,714/2,189	78
Negative tuberculin test	488/702	70	2,093/3,268	64
Hyperglobulinaemia	161/526	31	808/1,832	44
Hypercalcaemia	99/547	18	200/1,760	11
Total	818	100	3,676	100

Table 4–2. Percentage Frequency of Involvement of Various Tissues in Sarcoidosis, Based on a Worldwide Survey of 3,676 Patients*

	Intra Thoracic	Reticulo- Endothelial	Skin	Erythema Nodosum	Eyes	Parotid	CNS	Bone
London	84	41	25	31	27	6	7	4
New York	92	55	19	11	20	8	4	9
Paris	94	32	12	6.5	11	6	4	4.5
Los Angeles	93	46	27	9	11	6	2	4
Tokyo	87	24	12	4	32	5	4	2
Reading	89	30	13	32	16	5	9	1
Lisbon	88	29	18	12	6	2	4	13
Edinburgh	94	39	6.8	33	11	5	3	1.2
Novi Sad	90	14	4	11	15	2.5	1.4	11
Naples	99	0	0.4	6	0	0	0	0
Geneva	97	17	6	11	12	2	1	3
Total	87	28	9	17	15	4	4	3

*Reticulo-endothelial = peripheral lymphadenopathy and splenomegaly.

Table 4–3. Multisystem Modes of Presentation of Sarcoidosis

Ophthalmologist	Chest Physician	Dermatologist
Uveitis	Routine chest x-ray	Erythema nodosum
Uveo-parotitis	Breathlessness	Maculopapular eruptions
Sjögren's syndrome	Nasopharyngitis	Scars
Retinal vasculitis	Pulmonary fibrosis	Keloids
Papilloedema	Cor pulmonale	Lupus pernio
Choroidoretinitis		Plaques
Glaucoma		
Cataract		
Physician	**Neurologist**	**Biochemist**
PUO	Cranial nerve palsy	Hydroxyprolinuria
Enlarged parotids	Neuropathy	Hyperglobulinaemia
Lymphadenopathy	Myopathy	Hypercalcaemia
Splenomegaly	Meningitis	Hyperuricemia
Liver granulomas	Space-occupying lesions	Hypercalciuria
		Raised SACE
Cardiologist	**Urologist**	**Rheumatologist**
Cardiac arrhythmia	Hypercalciuria	Polyarthralgia
Bundle branch block	Renal calculi	Bone cysts
Cardiomyopathy	Nephrocalcinosis	Dactylitis
Heart block	Uraemia	Gout
Rheumatic fever–like symptoms		Acute rheumatism–like symptoms
Gastroenterologist	**Immunologist**	**Ear, Nose, Throat Surgeon**
Liver granulomas	Cutaneous energy	Collapsing nose
Splenomegaly	Lymphoproliferation	Nasal granulomas
Portal hypertension	OKT 4:T8 ratio	Nasal bone necrosis
Intrahepatic Cholestasis	High ESR	Laryngeal granulomas
Crohn's disease–like symptoms	Activated macrophages	Hoarseness
Whipple's disease–like symptoms	HLA/DRW profile	Croup
		Stridor

Table 4–4. Age at Presentation of Sarcoidosis in the Royal Northern Hospital Compared with the Worldwide Series*

	Royal Northern Hospital	Worldwide
Female	61	57
Caucasian	89	79
Black	10	10
Japanese	—	8
Decade of Presentation 0–40	74	68
41–60 +	26	32

*Expressed as percentages of the total series.

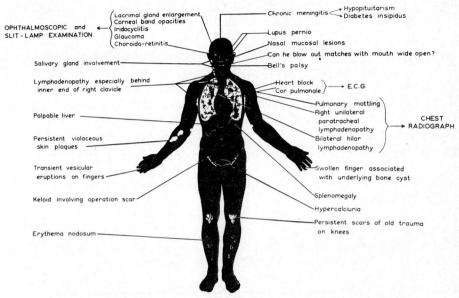

Figure 4–1. Clinical examination of a patient with suspected sarcoidosis.

INTRATHORACIC (see Chapter 5)

Only about 8 per cent of patients present and continue to have a normal chest x-ray. The majority present with bilateral hilar lymphadenopathy (51 per cent); the outcome is particularly favourable when the bilateral hilar lymphadenopathy is associated with erythema nodosum. The person with pulmonary sarcoidosis may also have skin or ocular lesions, reticulo-endo-thelial involvement, and possibly upper respiratory tract sarcoidosis.

Table 4–5. Age, Sex, and Race of 810 Patients with Sarcoidosis

Age of Onset	< 21	21–30	31–40	41–50	> 50	Total No.	%
Male	24	141	93	37	20	318*	39
Female	28	199	119	88	61	500*	61
English	39	244	140	103	71	597	74
W. Indian	5	23	33	14	4	79	10
Irish	4	39	13	4	3	63	8
Other	4	34	26	4	3	71	9
Overall Total	52	340	212	125	81	810	100

*Age of onset of eight patients unknown.

SARCOIDOSIS OF THE UPPER RESPIRATORY TRACT (see Chapter 5)

Sarcoidosis of the upper respiratory tract (SURT) involves the nose, nasopharyngeal mucosa, and larynx. It is frequently associated with lupus pernio and may, in fact, precede and herald the onset of lupus pernio, a fact which is of practical clinical importance. SURT is a chronic manifestation occurring twice as often in women as in men and usually presenting in the third decade, just as lupus pernio occurs much more commonly in women in the fourth and fifth decades of life. A clinically significant point is that SURT may present to the nose and throat surgeon, who may perform a submucous resection for relief of nasal symptoms, with disastrous results including nasal septal perforation and progressive destruction of bone and cartilaginous septum.

OCULAR INVOLVEMENT (see Chapter 6)

Slit-lamp examination of the eyes should be routine. Lesions include acute and chronic iridocyclitis, choroidoretinitis, papilloedema, keratoconjunctivitis, conjunctival follicles, and the late complications of cataracts and secondary glaucoma. Ocular involvement is one manifestation of a multisystem disorder in which many clinical associations are often interwoven into well-defined patterns of disease. Acute iritis, erythema nodosum, and hilar adenopathy have a benign self-limiting course and a satisfactory outcome. Lupus pernio is associated with chronic uveitis, pulmonary fibrosis, and bone cysts; the course is persistent and troublesome. Keratoconjunctivitis sicca, with or without parotid and lacrimal gland enlargement, mimics Sjögren's syndrome. Parotid gland enlargement, anterior uveitis, and facial palsy constitute Heerfordt's syndrome.

NEUROSARCOIDOSIS (see Chapter 6)

This occurs in about 4 to 7 per cent of patients with sarcoidosis. Facial palsy is the most frequent presentation, either alone or with other cranial nerve palsies or papilloedema. Other features include peripheral neuropathy, myopathy, meningitis, space-occupying brain lesions, epilepsy, cerebellar ataxia, hypopituitarism, and diabetes insipidus. Neurosarcoidosis has a mortality of 10 per cent, which is twice the overall mortality of sarcoidosis. The response to corticosteroids is more likely to occur in younger patients with an explosive onset of meningitis with erythema nodosum than in those with a space-occupying intracranial mass, chronic skin lesions, chronic uveitis, or pulmonary fibrosis.

SKIN LESIONS (see Chapter 7)

Erythema nodosum is associated with bilateral hilar lymphadenopathy, polyarthralgia, and occasionally acute iritis. It predominates in women of the child-bearing years and is often associated with pregnancy or lactation, suggesting a hormonal factor in its genesis. Transient circulating immune complexes may be detectable in this phase of sarcoidosis.

Lupus pernio is a chronic persistent violaceous lesion with a predilection for the nose, cheeks, and ears. It reflects chronic fibrotic sarcoidosis. It develops insidiously and progresses indolently over the years.

Other skin lesions include persistent plaques, maculopapular eruptions, scars, and keloids. These keloids may be found at the sites of surgery, ear piercing, tattooing, repeated venesection in the antecubital fossa, or even where tuberculin and other skin tests have been performed.

THE HEART (see Chapter 8)

Myocardial sarcoidosis is difficult to recognize clinically. It should be considered if a patient with florid multisystem sarcoidosis develops bundle branch block, arrhythmias, congestive cardiac failure, pericarditis, or clinical evidence of cardiomyopathy. Sudden death without previous evidence of a heart lesion may occur, particularly in patients over 40 years of age. Macroscopic changes are most evident in the posterior part of the ventricular septum. Microscopy discloses granulomas or fibrous tissue or an admixture.

LYMPHORETICULAR (see Chapter 9)

The lymph nodes and spleen were enlarged in 39 per cent of patients in the London series and in 28 per cent of patients worldwide. Hepatomegaly was noted in 82 (10 per cent) and hepatosplenomegaly in 43 (5 per cent).

LOCOMOTOR (see Chapter 10)

Bone sarcoidosis, a hallmark of chronic fibrotic sarcoidosis, was noted in 31 (4 per cent) patients in the London series and in 109 (3 per cent) patients worldwide. It is most frequent in the hands and feet and rarely may involve the temporal or frontal bone, the hard palate, and nasal cartilage. It is associated with soft tissue swelling, joint stiffness, and pain. There is no correlation between bone involvement and abnormal calcium metabolism. There are three radiological types of bone lesions:

1. Permeative: There is progressive cortical "tunnelling" with remodeling of trabecular and cortical architecture.

2. Lytic: These punched-out cysts are associated with pressure narrowing of the shaft, pathological fractures, and residual cavities.

3. Destructive: Rapid destructive change may cause secondary joint surface involvement, and this may be followed by a periosteal reaction.

Muscle disease runs a course independent from bone disease but may be just as troublesome. It comprises acute polymyositis, chronic myopathy, muscle nodules, contractures, and atrophy.

MISCELLANEOUS SITES

Kidney. Although hypercalcaemia has been noted in 99 of 547 (18 per cent) patients in whom it was sought, nephrocalcinosis with irreversible renal damage was only noted in 10 (1 per cent) patients (see Chapter 11).

Parotid Glands. These glands were enlarged in 52 (6 per cent) patients (see Chapter 11).

Lacrimal Gland. Enlargement of this gland was evident in 22 (2.6 per cent) patients (see Chapter 6).

TEN POINTERS TO CLINICAL MANAGEMENT

Sarcoidosis usually presents in the 20- to 40-year age group to the chest physician, ophthalmologist, or dermatologist. When confronted with suspected sarcoidosis, the following investigative routine is recommended:

1. Full general medical examination, including ophthalmoscopy.

2. Slit lamp examination of the eyes; otherwise, silent lesions may be overlooked.

3. Chest radiography.

4. Serum calcium level, which is elevated in up to 20 per cent of patients. It is also preferable to do routine 24-hour urine calcium levels; hypercalciuria may occur despite normal serum calcium levels.

5. Histological confirmation by fibreoptic bronchoscopy or biopsy of lymph node, skin, liver, minor salivary gland, gum, or muscle or Kveim-Siltzbach skin test.

6. Make sure that granulomas are multisystemic.

7. Serum angiotensin-converting enzyme level, which offers a monitor of progress of the disease (see Chapter 14).

8. Tuberculin skin test, which is negative in two-thirds of patients (see Chapter 13).

9. Special situations may call for fluorescein angiography for suspected posterior uveitis, radioactive thallium for evidence of myocardial involvement, CAT scanning for neurosarcoidosis, and radioactive gallium as a monitor of progress (see Chapters 6 and 14).

10. Judge whether the disease is acute or chronic. Lines of treatment depend on this crucial judgement (see Chapter 17).

COURSE AND PROGNOSIS

Dr. Neville analysed the prognostic factors in our series of 818 patients.[1] Disease outcome was assessed by chest x-ray resolution and by evidence of complete remission of sarcoidosis at two years. He produced a percentage prognostic index that showed the outcome of acute arthritis and erythema nodosum to be high and good and that of cor pulmonale to be low and poor. Other features fall between these extremes (Tables 4–6 and 4–7).

The natural history of sarcoidosis and the response to treatment vary with the type of disease. Since there is a high incidence of spontaneous remission, evaluation of any therapeutic regimen is difficult, for it must take into account the different behaviour and fate of these two forms—subacute (transient) and chronic (persistent) sarcoidosis (see Chapter 17). Undoubtedly the most predictable course and the best prognosis accompany erythema nodosum. It usually subsides within a month of onset (Fig. 4–2), and accompanying hilar adenopathy will regress in the course of one year (Fig. 4–3). Recurrence and sequelae are rare. Erythema nodosum is not an

Table 4–6. A Prognostic Index of Sarcoidosis Based on the Outcome of 818 Patients

Feature	Chest Resolution		Remission in Two Years		Prognostic Index*
	No.	%	*No.*	%	
Acute Arthritis	115/166	69	148/178	83	76
Erythema nodosum	147/231	64	210/251	84	74
Hilar lymphadenopathy	268/458	59	334/458	73	66
Irish	33/60	55	42/65	65	60
Female	243/426	57	307/500	61	59
Age < 31	178/350	51	254/392	65	58
Overall Intrathoracic	362/700	52	467/818	57	54
English	268/527	51	341/602	57	54
Age > 30	162/360	45	211/417	51	48
Peripheral adenopathy	85/185	46	109/220	50	48
Lacrimals	9/21	43	11/22	50	47
Ocular	99/215	46	105/224	47	46
Male	106/274	39	160/318	50	45
West Indian	25/72	35	43/79	54	45
BHL + infiltration	59/150	39	77/150	51	45
Parotid	21/43	49	15/52	29	39
Spleen	32/82	39	35/100	35	37
Pulmonary infiltration	35/92	38	31/92	34	36
Heart	3/9	33	3/9	33	33
Central nervous system	22/56	39	19/77	25	32
Hepatomegaly	21/65	32	22/82	27	29
Lupus pernio	7/24	29	5/33	15	22
Larynx	1/5	20	1/5	20	20
SURT	4/19	21	3/21	14	18
Bone	4/21	19	4/31	13	16
Nephrocalcinosis	1/9	11	0/10	0	5
Cor pulmonale	0/18	0	0/18	0	0

*Expressed as percentage; mean of resolution × remission.

Table 4–7. Prognosis of Sarcoidosis Based on Table 4–6

Good	Fair	Poor
Abrupt onset	Insidious onset	Insidious onset
Female	Male	Lupus pernio
< 30	> 30	SURT
English	West Indian	Bone cysts
Irish		Nephrocalcinosis
X Ray I	II/III	Cor pulmonale
Erythema nodosum	Lacrimals/parotids	
	Spleen/lymph nodes	
	Cardiac/CNS	

indication for steroid therapy because recovery is complete without it. It is often tempting to prescribe it for symptomatic relief in patients with hectic fever and severe polyarthralgia. Nevertheless, it is possible that steroids may interfere with some important immune mechanisms of which we are at present ignorant. It seems unneccessary to prescribe such potent drugs for such a benign self-limiting condition.

It is not possible, unfortunately, to define such a clear-cut natural history in other forms of sarcoidosis, except to predict that maculopapular eruptions, conjunctivitis, salivary gland enlargement, Bell's palsy, and peripheral lymphadenopathy usually regress without treatment in the course of one year. On the other hand, chronic iridocyclitis, keratoconjunctivitis sicca, lupus pernio, plaques, and keloids persist unchanged or with minor fluctuations indefinitely.

Skin and pulmonary lesions follow a very similar course and likewise parallel each other's response to treatment. Trransient skin lesions are usually associated with hilar adenopathy, whereas chronic skin lesions are more likely to be accompanied by pulmonary fibrosis. The former tend to clear without treatment, whereas the latter fail to do so despite prolonged corticosteroid therapy. Resolution of all types of pulmonary sarcoidosis may be expected in two-thirds of patients. It is less likely to be achieved in older

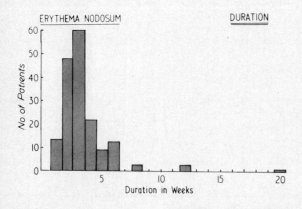

Figure 4–2. Erythema nodosum usually subsides within one month.

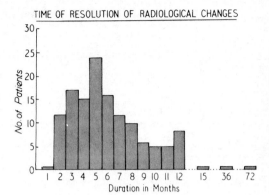

Figure 4–3. Hilar adenopathy regresses within one year.

patients and in those in whom there is accompanying extrathoracic disease, particularly bone and skin lesions (Fig. 4–4). The combination of pulmonary and cutaneous sarcoidosis constitutes the hallmark of chronicity, presumably because longstanding fibrosis has supervened. Clearing of the abnormal chest x-ray occurred in only one-third of patients with bone cysts, one-fifth with skin lesions, and one-sixth of patients in whom bone and skin lesions accompanied pulmonary sarcoidosis.

Sarcoidosis would remain a relatively benign and unimportant disease but for the development of certain devastating complications due to the irreversible fibrosis in the lungs and eyes and abnormal calcium metabolism affecting the kidneys (Table 4–8).

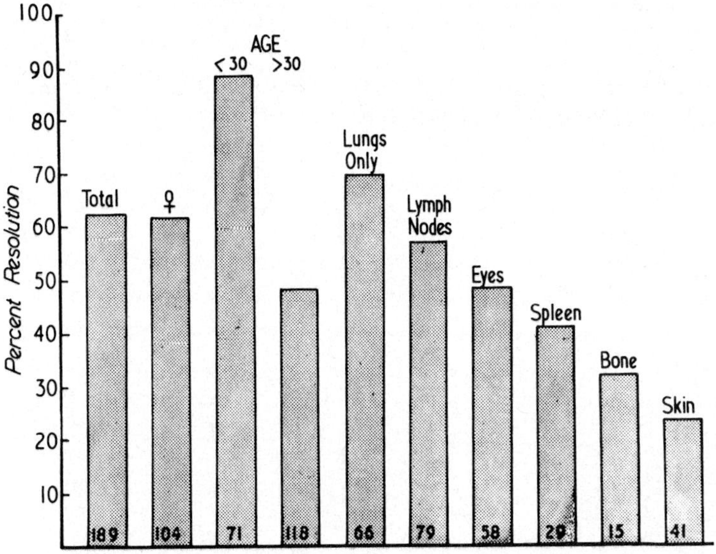

Figure 4–4. Resolution of pulmonary sarcoidosis is less likely if there are bone and skin lesions, which are the hallmarks of chronicity.

Table 4–8. Complications of Sarcoidosis

Clinical Features	Complications	Failure of
Pulmonary fibrosis	Cor pulmonale	Lungs Heart
Chronic uveitis	Glaucoma, cataract	Vision
Hypercalcaemia Hypercalciuria	Nephrocalcinosis	Kidneys

In assessing the prognosis, it is important to assess the degree of functional failure of lungs, heart, eyes, and kidneys. In the practical management of sarcoidosis, it is the physician's duty to diagnose the condition sufficiently early so that the judicious use of corticosteroids may prevent these unfortunate sequelae. In fact, the main indications for corticosteroid therapy are directed toward this goal. Steroids should be prescribed when there is ocular involvement or worsening or static pulmonary involvement and to reverse persistent hypercalciuria. By way of contrast there is no absolute indication for treating skin lesions, since no disabling sequelae are anticipated. Chronic fibrotic lesions are less likely to respond than are fresh active sarcoid lesions. Recurrence may follow cessation of treatment. With these two principles in mind, it may be added that skin lesions that are not unsightly do not warrant the transient benefits of treatment (see Chapter 7).

REFERENCE

1. Neville E, Walker A N, James D G. Prognostic factors predicting the outcome of sarcoidosis: An analysis of 818 patients. Quart J Med 208:525, 1983.

5

Intrathoracic and Upper Respiratory Tract

INTRODUCTION

It would seem natural, in a discussion of respiratory tract sarcoidosis, to commence with the upper respiratory tract and then consider the lower tract. In fact, the lung is traditionally discussed first because it is far more frequently involved and sarcoidosis of the upper respiratory tract (SURT) has only received attention more recently. Furthermore, they are strange bedfellows and bear little relationship to each other, although they both constitute the same tract. Intrathoracic involvement is evident in nine-tenths of patients, whereas SURT was noted in 53 of 818 (6 per cent) patients in this series.

INTRATHORACIC TRACT

The paucity of symptoms despite widespread radiographical changes distinguishes sarcoidosis from other diseases such as extrinsic allergic alveolitis and chronic beryllium disease. Cough is an infrequent feature, and wheezing or bronchospasm points to segmental bronchial narrowing (see page 58). Breathlessness suggests irreversible chronic fibrotic disease, and haemoptysis also indicates this late stage with secondary *Aspergillus* infection or cavitation or both. Pleurisy, pleural effusions, and finger clubbing are so infrequent that they should increase the probability of another diagnosis. Spontaneous pneumothorax is a rare complication of the late stage of chronic fibrotic sarcoidosis.

STAGES

It is customary to stage intrathoracic sarcoidosis according to these chest x-ray changes on first presentation:

Stage 0—clear chest radiograph
Stage 1—hilar lymphadenopathy (Fig. 5–1A)
Stage 2—hilar lymphadenopathy and pulmonary infiltration (Fig. 5–2A)
Stage 3—pulmonary infiltration without hilar adenopathy (Fig. 5–3A)

49

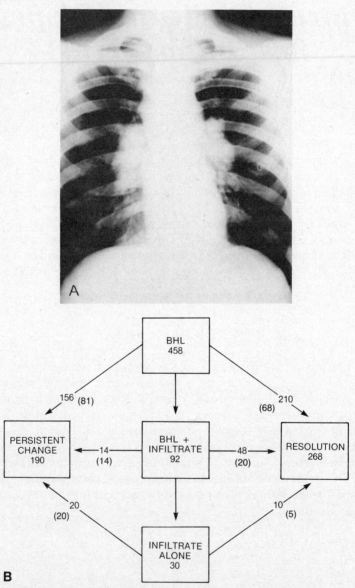

Figure 5–1. *A*, Hilar adenopathy. *B*, Chest x-ray changes of bilateral hilar lymphadenopathy seen with resolution or persistent change. Numbers in parentheses represent patients treated with steroids.

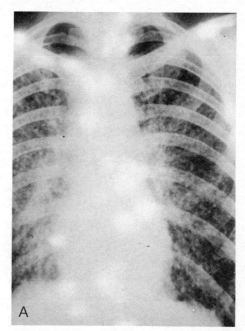

Figure 5–2. A, Hilar adenopathy and pulmonary infiltration. B, Flow patterns of the chest x-ray changes of patients presenting with a Stage 2 chest x-ray abnormality. As in Figure 5–1B, numbers in parentheses represent patients treated with steroids.

A

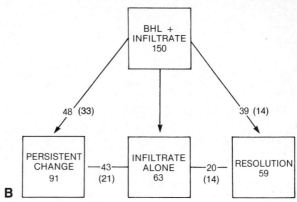

B

This is a crude classification with much overlapping. Lung biopsy may unexpectedly reveal sarcoid granulomas in Stages 0 and 1. Stage 3 may be an indivisible radiological mixture of irreversible fibrosis and reversible granulomas. Allowing for many shortcomings, this staging is simple, and, most importantly, it is recognised and understood throughout the world. Some centres make refinements, such as adding Stage 4; this suggests an even more advanced stage than Stage 3, with more irreversible fibrosis and perhaps evidence of complicating cor pulmonale.

We have compared the chest x-ray changes on presentation and the fate of patients in a homogeneous Royal Northern Hospital series with those observed in a heterogeneous worldwide survey (Table 5–1).

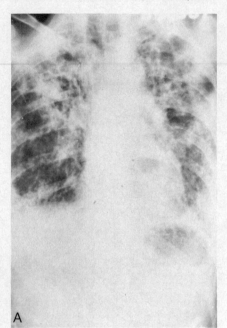

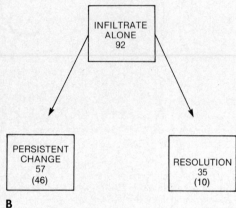

```
          ┌─────────────┐
          │  INFILTRATE │
          │    ALONE    │
          │     92      │
          └─────────────┘
           ↙           ↘
┌─────────────┐      ┌─────────────┐
│ PERSISTENT  │      │             │
│   CHANGE    │      │ RESOLUTION  │
│     57      │      │     35      │
│    (46)     │      │    (10)     │
└─────────────┘      └─────────────┘
B
```

Figure 5–3. *A*, Pulmonary infiltration. *B*, Prognosis of patients presenting with a Stage 3 chest x-ray change. Numbers in parentheses represent patients treated with steroids

A

Table 5–1. Intrathoracic Involvement and Eventual Resolution Worldwide and in the Royal Northern Hospital Series

Features	Worldwide Series		Royal Northern Hospital Series	
	No.	*%*	*No.*	*%*
Stage at presentation				
0	277	8	118	13
1	1,865	51	458	65
2	1,066	29	150	22
3	446	12	92	13
Total	3,654	100	818	100
Eventual chest x-ray resolution				
1	1,217	65	268	59
2	490	46	59	39
3	90	20	35	38
Overall resolution	1,797	49	362	52

Stage 1

Hilar adenopathy was bilateral in all but 20 patients who presented with unilateral hilar adenopathy. There was eventual resolution in 268 of 458 (59 per cent) patients (see Table 5–1), but there were various courses before this was achieved (see Fig. 5–1). This resolution occurred directly in 210 but with infiltration in 58 instances.

Steroid therapy did not seem to influence resolution, for it was given to two-thirds of those who failed to resolve and only to one-third of those who did attain chest x-ray resolution (Table 5–2). The chances of achieving a clear chest x-ray sooner or later in the London Series (59 per cent) are similar to those of other world centres (65 per cent).

Stage 2

One hundred-fifty patients presented at this later stage and only 59 (39 per cent) eventually achieved a clear chest radiograph (see Fig. 5–2). Once again steroid therapy did not seem to improve the incidence of resolution, for it was used with equal frequency in those who did and did not achieve resolution (see Table 5–2). Here again the incidence of resolution in the London series is similar to that in the worldwide survey (46 per cent).

Stage 3

This is a late stage of presentation and it spells chronicity and pulmonary fibrosis, for resolution only occurred in 38 per cent (see Fig. 5–3 and Table 5–2). Steroid therapy seemed to be singularly ineffective (see Table 5–2).

A French school subdivides the radiological changes of pulmonary sarcoidosis into three types of diffuse interstitial opacities—reticular, reticulo-

Table 5–2. Influence of Steroid Therapy on Each Stage of Intrathoracic Involvement and Resolution*

Chest X-ray Stage	Number of Patients	Steroid Therapy		Outcome in 362 Patients Achieving Chest X-ray Resolution			
				Without Steroids		With Steroids	
		No.	%	No.	%	No.	%
1	458	208	45	175	65	93	35
2	150	82	55	31	53	28	47
3	92	56	61	25	71	10	29
Total	700	346	49	231	63	131	37

*Data from Neville E, Walker AM, James DG. Prognostic factors predicting the outcome of sarcoidosis: An analysis of 818 patients. Quart J Med. New Series L11, 208:525, 1983.

micronodular, and nodular (nodules less than 5 mm in diameter).[1] Less frequently the radiological pattern is called *alveolar*. Whereas reticular patterns are liable to persist, alveolar sarcoidosis has an acute course and disappears even without steroids.

Influence of Steroid Therapy on Chest X-Ray Resolution

Oral steroids were given to 208 (45 per cent) patients with Stage 1 involvement, 82 (55 per cent) with Stage 2 changes, and 56 (61 per cent) with Stage 3 disease. Of the 700 patients with a chest x-ray abnormality, complete radiological resolution was eventually achieved in 362 (52 per cent) (see Table 5–1); one-third achieved radiological resolution with steroids and two-thirds without steroids (see Table 5–2). Although there was no evidence that steroid therapy influenced the resolution of chest x-ray changes in pulmonary sarcoidosis, it is possible that without this therapy the number of patients with chronic persistent disease and its attendant morbidity might have been greater. Moreover, steroid therapy certainly provided symptomatic relief from disabling breathlessness and overcame many manifestations of extrathoracic sarcoidosis.

The US Army has also made a long-term follow-up study, which fails to show any benefit at 6 months, at 1 to 2 years, and at 10 to 15 years.[2]

The considerable experience at the Johns Hopkins Hospital (1960 to 1975) may be summarised as follows:

. . . Benefits coincident with corticosteroid treatment are demonstrated and worsening frequently occurs when treatment is withdrawn. This provides strong support for the beneficial effects of corticosteroid treatment in active symptomatic pulmonary sarcoidosis. The benefits accrued far exceed the problems encountered.[3]

BRONCHO-ALVEOLAR LAVAGE (BAL)

The ability to sample the secretions of the lower respiratory tract by fibreoptic bronchoscopy has improved our understanding of interstitial and granulomatous lung diseases.[4-6]

About 100 to 300 ml of 0.9% saline is instilled in four to six aliquots and retrieved by suction. This provides specimens for alveolar macrophages and lymphocytes, T and B cells, lysozyme, angiotensin-converting enzyme (ACE) complement, proteins, and immunoglobulins. With any interpretation of the results, it is important to know whether the patient is a smoker, for this doubles the yield of cells and increases ACE threefold and lysozyme twofold. Sarcoidosis is characterised by an increase of T helper cells and alveolar macrophages, and there is also a non-specific increase of IgG-secreting cells. The levels of these various constituents of BAL do not correlate closely with

Table 5–3. Broncho-alveolar Lavage as a Means of Distinguishing
Sarcoidosis and Idiopathic Pulmonary Fibrosis*

Cells	Sarcoidosis	Idiopathic Pulmonary Fibrosis
Macrophages	Decreased	Decreased
T helper	Marked increase	Normal
T suppressor	Marked decrease	Normal
B cell	Decreased	Normal
Neutrophils	Normal	Marked increase
Eosinophils	± Increase	Increase
Basophils	± Increase	± Increase

*Based on Rossi AG, Hunninghake GW, Crystal RG. Evaluation of inflammatory and immune processes in the interstitial lung disorders: Use of bronchoalveolar lavage. *In* Cumming G, Bonsignore G (eds): Cellular Biology of the Lung. Plenum Press, New York. p 107, 1982.

blood levels, and they presumably reflect activated alveolar macrophage activity.

BAL is a helpful marker of activity of sarcoidosis, and serial determinations monitor the progress and response to treatment. Alveolar ACE is a more sensitive marker than serum ACE (SACE),[7] but it is, of course, far easier to monitor progress with SACE. BAL is not helpful in distinguishing sarcoidosis from other granulomatous lung disorders, including hypersensitivity pneumonitis, but it is helpful in distinguishing it from idiopathic pulmonary fibrosis at a stage when both have considerable alveolitis (Table 5–3).[8]

PULMONARY PATHOLOGY

Non-caseating epithelioid cell granulomas are found in the interstitium (Fig. 5–4), predominantly in the upper two-thirds of the lungs and conspicuous in the fixed parts—subpleural, septal, peri- and intrabronchial, and peri- and intravascular. Granulomas are discrete and only just visible to the naked eye but may coalesce with associated fibrosis to form palpable "conglomerate" nodules up to 3 cm in diameter.[9] Granulomas involving small pulmonary vessels are well-recognised, but primary vascular diseases need to be excluded (see page 61). Involvement of large pulmonary arteries has also been reported,[10] but it should not be confused with Wegener's granulomatosis. Involvement of the bronchial wall may result in stenosis and may contribute to the deformities seen in chronic disease (Fig. 5–5).

Based on BAL studies,[11, 12] alveolitis is claimed to be of prime importance and of prognostic significance; high-intensity alveolitis signifies deteriorating function and is an indication for therapy. There also seems to be an inverse

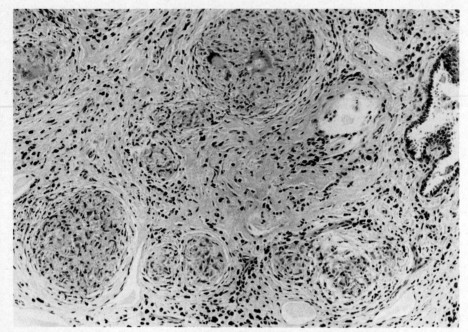

Figure 5–4. Discrete pulmonary interstitial epithelioid cell granulomas. H & E × 80.

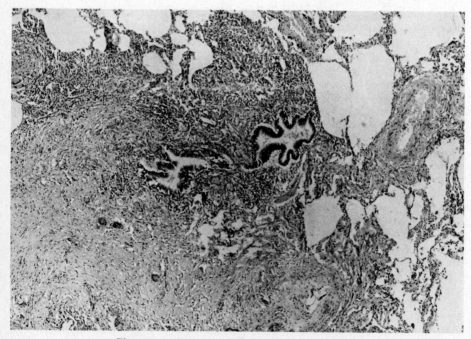

Figure 5–5. Bronchial wall stenosis. H & E × 50.

relationship between alveolitis and granuloma formation. These claims should become more secure when there is an accurate comparison between BAL and tissue examination, but this is not always available. Alveolitis is inconspicuous in sarcoidosis compared with chronic beryllium disease[13] (CBD) and acute farmer's lung[14] (AFL).

The granulomas of sarcoidosis tend to be more frequent in the upper parts of the lung. Inclusion bodies are very frequent, and the granulomas persist in the presence of developing fibrosis. CBD and AFL mimic sarcoidosis very closely, so that prominent alveolitis becomes a most important distinctive feature. Granulomas in CBD may show considerable necrosis, which may be related to dose and hypersensitivity.[15] The predominant centrilobular distribution of granulomas in AFL reflect the port of entry of the causative antigen and along with alveolitis are very useful diagnostic features. It should also be noted that granulomas in AFL are transient and, strangely, disappear completely in the chronic fibrotic phase of the disease.

In about 10 per cent of sarcoidosis patients, the granulomas persist with the development of extensive, patchy fibrosis, mainly affecting the upper and middle lobes. There is frequently associated bronchiectasis, bronchiolectasis, and cystic, honeycomb changes (Fig. 5–6).

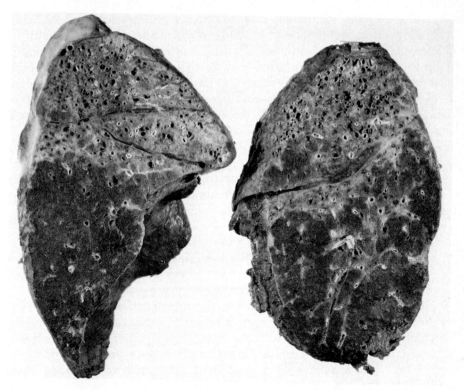

Figure 5–6. Right and left lungs revealing upper zone diffuse fibrosis with honeycomb change. × 0.50.

The granulomas of miliary tuberculosis are very widely disseminated and may show necrosis, and culture will reveal the causative organism.

Clinical pleural involvement, effusion, and pneumothorax are rare.[16] Pneumothorax may result from ruptured cysts. Emphysema is not a feature of sarcoidosis, and we have no evidence to support the suggestion that granulomas rupture directly into the pleura.

BRONCHOSTENOSIS[17, 18]

We have noted stridor due to laryngeal involvement and expiratory bronchospasm associated with bronchostenosis. Fibreoptic bronchoscopy reveals bronchial mucosal involvement due to lobar or segmental bronchostenosis. There may be multiple segmental stenoses associated with an asthma-like clinical picture and evidence of mixed restrictive and obstructive defects in pulmonary function tests. Steroid therapy is certainly indicated in an attempt to overcome the bronchospasm, but the response is mixed, as might be expected at this late stage of bronchial fibrosis.

Although rare, it would not be surprising to find localised bronchial narrowing in patients with widespread end-stage pulmonary fibrosis. It is surprising, but also fortunately rare, to observe multiple localised bronchial narrowings at bronchoscopy at an early stage of the disease and with no radiographical evidence of pulmonary fibrosis. If a patient develops sudden breathlessness or wheezing, then it is worth supplementing bronchoscopy with bronchography. At the time of fibreoptic bronchoscopy, aqueous propyliodone is used to outline bronchial narrowing, which may not be visualised on bronchoscopy alone. Cicatricial fibrosis seen at the late stages seems unlikely at this early stage. We do not know whether narrowing is due to granulomas with considerable oedema or to an accelerated stage of fibrosis. The response to steroid therapy would suggest the latter, for the response is not one of dramatic, permanent improvement. There is some clinical improvement, but lung function abnormalities persist and long-term therapy is necessary.

PHYSIOLOGY

Pulmonary sarcoidosis is characterised by a restrictive defect, an impaired transfer factor (T_LCO), and a lowered transfer co-efficient (KCO). The response of KCO to exercise is a more sensitive index of changed function than more routine pulmonary function tests. There are discrepancies between the chest radiograph and routine lung function tests because pulmonary granulomas and alveolitis may occur in the presence of a normal chest radiograph. The impairment of lung function depends on the size and number of pulmonary granulomas and their location. The primary value of the exercise KCO test is that it reveals impairment even in the presence of an apparently normal chest radiograph.[19]

Airflow obstruction in small airways is also present more frequently than had been realised by routine spirometry. In one series, nearly three-fourths of patients had some evidence of airflow obstruction.[20] Of these, about three-fifths had small airways abnormalities and one-tenth had flow rate reduction due to loss of elastic recoil. Yet again, there was no significant correlation between the abnormal lung function and the chest x-ray appearance. With increasing pulmonary infiltration, there is a reduction of vital capacity, airway resistance, maximum mid-expiratory flow, and arterial oxygen tension on exercise. The worse the pretreatment impairment, the greater the immediate response to corticosteroid therapy, both clinically and in these tests of lung function. However, this is illusory, for with reduction or cessation of treatment there is usually a return of the functional abnormalities.

Airway hyper-reactivity also plays a role in some patients, as demonstrated by bronchoprovocation testing with a methacholine challenge. Sarcoid patients with increased reactivity had more airway obstruction, smaller vital capacity, lower single-breath diffusing capacity for carbon monoxide, and more wheezing and coughing.[21]

An obstructive defect may be demonstrated by flow-volume loops at a time when the lungs are radiologically clear.[22]

POSITRON TOMOGRAPHY[23]

Regional extravascular lung density and blood volume have been measured by positron emission tomography. Lung density was measured in units of gm/ml of thoracic volume, using an external ring source containing positron emitting ^{68}Be/^{68}Ga. Blood volume was measured after labelling circulating red cells with inhaler ^{11}CO. Extravascular lung density was obtained by subtracting blood volume from lung density. Radiographs were scored with a semiquantitative technique. All sarcoidosis patients showed increased extravascular lung density, and there was an inverse correlation between it and transfer factor (T_LCO/VA). Regional blood volume was slightly reduced. Steroid therapy led to improvement in the chest radiograph and lung function tests, and some patients showed a marked reduction in extravascular lung density.

DIFFERENTIAL DIAGNOSIS

There are numerous conditions that mimic pulmonary sarcoidosis (Tables 5–4 and 5–5), so it is essential to obtain histological confirmation of the diagnosis. This is most easily obtained by fibreoptic bronchoscopy;

Table 5–4. Radiological Differential Diagnosis of Intrathoracic Sarcoidosis

Stage	Type	Differential Diagnosis
1	Hilar lymphadenopathy	Hodgkin's disease Tuberculosis Metastases Pulmonary arteries Leukaemia Enlarged pulmonary arteries Infectious mononucleosis
2	Hilar adenopathy and pulmonary infiltration	Tuberculosis Pneumoconiosis Lymphangitic carcinoma Idiopathic haemosiderosis Pulmonary eosinophilia Alveolar cell carcinoma Histiocytosis-X
3	Diffuse pulmonary infiltration	As for Stage 2 *plus* Chronic beryllium disease Honeycomb lung Rheumatoid lung Progressive systemic sclerosis Rare pulmonary granulomatoses Fibrosing alveolitis Haemosiderosis Idiopathic fibrosis Carcinomatosis Sjögren's syndrome Extrinsic allergic alveolitis

flexible forceps biopsy is commendable for it yields both bronchial and lung tissue. A wide variety of techniques is available to suit the interests of all disciplines (see Chapter 3). Broncho-alveolar lavage (BAL) is helpful in the overall differential diagnosis, but it has not yet been sufficiently refined to differentiate one granulomatous lung disorder from another.

Chemical Lung Granulomas

There are three disorders due to granuloma-forming chemicals: beryllium disease, silicosis, and pulmonary talc granulomatosis.

Beryllium is a potent chemical sensitiser used increasingly in a variety of modern, predominantly metallurgical, industries.[13] A number of features (Table 5–6) are of value in distinguishing chronic beryllium disease from sarcoidosis, but without an occupational history mistakes are easily made, particularly as the disease may develop up to 20 years after exposure (Jones Williams, 1983). The *in vitro* beryllium lymphocyte transformation test authoritatively distinguishes beryllium disease from sarcoidosis, as it is always positive in beryllium patients and negative in patients with sarcoidosis.[24] It is likely that other industrial materials may produce a sarcoid-like illness. The granuloma of beryllium disease is indistinguishable from that of sarcoidosis.[13]

Table 5–5. Differential Diagnosis of Granulomatous Lung Diseases

Features	Wegener's Granulomatosis — Classic	Wegener's Granulomatosis — Limited	Lymphomatoid Granulomatosis	Churg-Strauss Syndrome	Necrotising Sarcoid Granulomatosis	Bronchocentric Granulomatosis — Asthma	Bronchocentric Granulomatosis — No Asthma	Sarcoidosis
F:M	M > F	Equal	M slightly more frequent	Same	Same	Same	Same	Same
Decade of age incidence	50	50	30–50	50	30 and 40	30	60	30 and 40
Presentation	Sinusitis Rhinorrhoea Epistaxis	+	Cough Dyspnoea Haemoptysis Arthralgia	Bronchitis Asthma Pneumonia	Fever Cough Pleurisy Malaise	Asthma	Cough Pleurisy Dyspnoea	Insignificant symptoms
Ulcerated nose and nasal septum	+	+	+	–	–	Bronchiectasis Bronchial obstruction Eosinophilia	–	Only when associated with lupus pernio and SURT
Saddle nose	+	+	–	–	–		–	
Chest x-ray — Opacities	+	+	+	+	+	Particularly in upper lobes	Particularly in upper lobes	+
Chest x-ray — Cavitation	+ +	+ +	+	Infiltration	+	Pulmonary fibrosis	Pulmonary fibrosis	Infiltration
Hilar adenopathy	–	–	–	–		–	–	+
Kidneys	Glomerulo-nephritis in 85%	–	Renal vasculitis	–		–	–	Nephro-calcinosis
Ocular	+	–	–	–	–	–	–	+
Allergy	±	±	–	+	–	+	±	–
Skin lesions	+ +	–	+ +	–	–	–	+	+ +
CNS	+ +	–	+ +	Rare	Rare	–	–	
Cardiac	+ +	–	–	–	–	–	–	
Characteristics	ESR ↑	–	–	Eosinophilia		Hypersensitivity to *aspergillus* Eosinophilia	Hypersensitivity to *aspergillus*	Raised SACE
Granulomas	±	±	Very rare	Infrequent	Always	+	+	Always
Vasculitis	+ +	+ +	Always	Always	+ +	±	±	Inconspicuous
Necrosis	Prominent and resemble infarcts	+ +	Prominent	Prominent	Prominent	+	+	Inconspicuous
Treatment	Cyclophosphamide		Cyclo-phosphamide Azathioprine	Steroids Azathioprine	Steroids Azathioprine	Corticosteroids	Corticosteroids	Steroids Azathioprine
Prognosis	Poor	Poor	Poor	Poor	Good	Good	Good	Good

+ = present; + + = prominent; – = absent; ± = inconspicuous.

Table 5–6. Features Distinguishing Sarcoidosis
and Chronic Beryllium Disease

Feature	Sarcoidosis	Chronic Beryllium Disease
Occupational exposure	No	Metal/alloy/ceramics
Onset	Acute or insidious	Insidious
Granuloma	Non-caseating	Rarely necrotic
Schaumann's bodies	70%	80%
Pulmonary fibrosis	10%	100%
Respiratory symptoms	Minimal	Moderate
Erythema nodosum	Frequent	No
Skin lesions	14%	Inoculation ulcer only
Bilateral hilar lymphadenopathy	Frequent	Rare
Uveitis	27%	Very rare
Bone cysts	3%	No
Skin tests		
Tuberculin	Negative in 66%	Normal
Kveim	Positive in 80%	Negative
Beryllium	Negative	Positive
Beryllium lymphocyte transformation test	Negative	Positive in 100%
Immune complexes	Positive in 50%	No
Raised SACE	60%	Rare
Genetic background	B8/A1/CW7/DR3	Not recognized
Prognosis	Good	Progressive fibrosis

Silicosis, following inhalation of pure silica, is rarely a problem in differential diagnosis, as the majority of patients radiologically show very dense nodular and rarely diffuse pulmonary fibrosis. Hilar lymphadenopathy is not a feature, and extrathoracic lesions rare. Silica and silicate granulomas are readily identified by the finding of crystalline birefringent crystals in macrophages with foreign body rather than Langhans-type giant cells.

Pulmonary talc granulomatosis is due to the inhalation or intravenous administration of talc. We have seen, as an incidental finding at autopsy, a patient with chronic rheumatoid arthritis who inhaled two to three packs of talcum powder a day. Both lungs showed innumerable sarcoid-like granulomas full of talc crystals but no evidence of interstitial fibrosis (Fig. 5–7). The similarity to sarcoidosis has been recently emphasised by six patients who developed pulmonary talc granulomas following long continued intravenous use of pentazocine (75% talc). These patients all showed raised SACE levels, positive gallium scans, and increased numbers of BAL lymphocytes. The diagnosis was established by the finding of talc crystals in the miliary pulmonary granulomas and in the broncho-alveolar washings.[25] Measurement is of value in distinguishing injected (average size 14.7 μm) from inhaled crystals (average size 3.57 μm).[26]

Extrinsic Allergic Alveolitis (EAA)

An increasing number of inhaled antigens, usually organic, are being recognised as a cause of antigen-antibody–induced lung disease in which

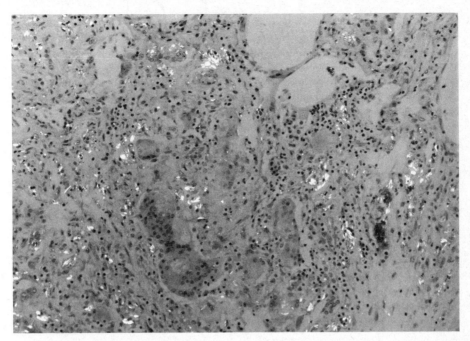

Figure 5–7. Pulmonary talcosis. Birefringent crystals within macrophages and giant cells. H & E × 80 (polarised light).

identical sarcoid granulomas may be present (Table 5–7). The essential basis for distinction from sarcoidosis is a history of exposure, environmental and often occupational, prominent alveolitis (Fig. 5–8), the presence of circulating antibodies to the causative antigens, and a negative Kveim-Siltzbach skin test.[14]

Other features distinguishing sarcoidosis from the commonest example of this group, acute farmer's lung disease, are erythema nodosum, bilateral hilar lymphadenopathy, uveitis, and various immunological abnormalities. Although antibodies and immune complexes have been shown in both exposed subjects and diseased patients, the levels in some patients with bird fancier's lung are reputed to be higher than those in healthy exposed subjects; thus antibodies indicate exposure but not necessarily disease.

The granulomas of EAA are very similar to those of sarcoidosis, but Schaumann's bodies are rare. In the chronic stage of EAA, somewhat surprisingly, the granulomas disappear without leaving small, round hyalinised scars, which are the hallmark of sarcoidosis.

Histiocytosis-X

The term *histiocytosis-X* encompasses a group of syndromes with diverse clinical features but a common denominator of granuloma formation with infiltration and proliferation of histiocytes. The clinical syndromes include

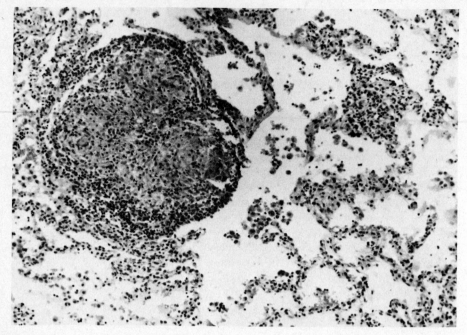

Figure 5–8. Acute farmer's lung. Sarcoid granulomas and prominent alveolitis. H & E × 80.

the fulminant Letterer-Siwe disease of early infancy, childhood Hand-Schüller-Christian disease, and in adult life a more benign, chronic form of the disorder, which may be confused with sarcoidosis (Table 5–8). It occurs in adult males, age 20 to 40, who present with respiratory symptoms, finger clubbing, recurrent pneumothorax, diabetes insipidus, and widespread pulmonary infiltration with cystic changes. The immunology is of considerable interest, for there is a notable lack of histamine H2 surface receptors on the T cells, suggesting a suppressor cell deficiency. This defect was corrected *in vitro* by incubation of the patient's lymphocytes with a crude extract of calf thymus gland. When this extract was given as a daily intramuscular injection to patients with histiocytosis-X, their immunological abnormalities were corrected and clinical remission resulted.[27]

Histiocytosis-X is distinguished from sarcoidosis by the clinicoradiographical features and also by the negative Kveim test and normal SACE levels (Table 5–9.) Histiocytosis-X shows a mixed cellular exudate, including foam cells, eosinophils, and characteristic X bodies in macrophages.[28, 29] X or Langerhans' bodies are an ultrastructural feature in 90 per cent of patients; they are identical to the granules in Langerhans' cells of the epidermis. They consist of intracytoplasmic rod-, plate-, or cup-like pentalaminar structures, which are diagnostic for histiocytosis-X (Fig. 5–9).

Table 5–7. Nature and Sources of Organic Dust Antigens in Extrinsic Allergic Alveolitis (Hypersensitivity Pneumonitis)*

Disease	Dust Exposure	Nature or Antigen to Which Precipitin Shown
Farmer's lung	Mouldy overheated hay	*Micropolyspora faeni* *Thermoactinomyces vulgaris*
Bagassosis	Mouldy overheated sugar cane bagasse	*Thermomycete sacchari*
Mushroom picker's lung	Mushroom compost dust	Thermophilic actinomycetes/ mushroom spores
Maltworker's lung	Mouldy barley or malt	*Aspergillus clavatus*
Bird fancier's lung	Pigeon and budgerigar droppings	Avian serum protein antigens
Pituitary snufftaker's lung	Powder of porcine and bovine posterior pituitary extract	Serum protein and pituitary antigens
Wheat weevil disease	Infested wheat flour	*Sitophilus granarius*
Maple stripper's lung	Infested maple bark	*Cryptostroma (Coniosporium) corticale*
Sequoisis	Mouldy redwood sawdust	*Aureobasidium (Pullularia) pullulans* *Graphium pullularia*
Suberosis	Cork dust	*Polyspora frequenta*
Woodworker's lung	Sawdusts of oak, cedar, etc.	Moulds
Cheese washer's lung	Moulds on cheese	*Penicillin* species
Paprika splitter's lung	Paprika	
Humidifier or air conditioner lung	Contaminated forced air system	Protozoa/amoebae

*Revised by Dr. John Edwards.

Table 5–8. Differences Between Sarcoidosis and Extrinsic Allergic Alveolitis

Feature	Sarcoidosis	Extrinsic Allergic Alveolitis/Hypersensitivity Pneumonitis
Histology	Identical	
Granulomas distribution	Widespread	Centrilobular
Interstitial pneumonitis	Mild	Prominent
Schaumann's bodies	70%	5%
Occupational history	No	Yes
Multisystem	Always	Sometimes
Erythema nodosum	Common	Absent
Hilar adenopathy	Frequent	Very rare
Wheezing	Rare	Common
Uveitis	Frequent	Absent
Depression of delayed type hypersensitivity	Yes	Yes
Circulating precipitins	Absent	Present
Raised or abnormal immunoglobulins	Yes	Yes
Kveim-Siltzbach test	Positive	Negative
Serum angiotensin-converting enzyme	Raised	Normal
Abnormal calcium metabolism	Frequent	Absent
Response to steroids	Good	Good
Prognosis	Good	Good if removed from exposure to antigen

Table 5–9. Features Distinguishing Sarcoidosis from Histiocytosis-X

Feature	Sarcoidosis	Histiocytosis-X
Male:female	Equal	4:1
Histology	Granulomas	Foam cells/eosinophils Langerhans' bodies
Multisystem	Yes	Yes
Bilateral hilar lymphadenopathy	Yes	No
Erythema nodosum	Yes	No
Bone cysts	Rare	More common
Depression delayed–type hypersensitivity	Usual	Uncommon
Kveim-Siltzbach test	Positive	Negative
Serum angiotensin-converting enzyme	Raised	Normal
Treatment	Steroids	Steroids/immunosuppressants
Prognosis	Good	Poor

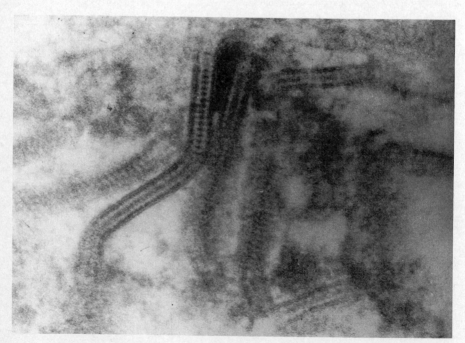

Figure 5–9. X bodies in macrophage of histiocytosis-X. EM × 50,000.

Other Granulomatous Lung Diseases

There are some other rare pulmonary granulomatoses that need to be distinguished from sarcoidosis,[30] including necrotising sarcoidal granulomatosis (NSG), Wegener's granulomatosis (WG), Churg-Strauss granulomatosis (CSG), bronchocentric granulomatosis (BCG), and lymphomatoid granulomatosis (LYG) (see Table 5–5).

Necrotising sarcoidal granulomatosis is of particular interest as being most likely to be confused with sarcoidosis. It has a similar good prognosis but differs in a number of important features. It is confined to the lungs with an absence of hilar lymphadenopathy. The majority of granulomas show conspicuous necrosis and particularly involve vessels and bronchi (Fig. 5–10). In a study of a recent case, for the first time we had evidence of a negative Kveim test, which strongly suggests that NSG is a separate entity and not a variant of sarcoidosis.[31]

All the other examples show major clinical and histological differences, in particular the rarity or absence of true focal sarcoid granulomas. WG[32] and CSG[33] are commonly associated with glomerulonephritis and show prominent tissue eosinophilia. WG often results in cavitating pulmonary infarcts (Fig. 5–11) and CSG with asthma. CSG often overlaps with polyarteritis nodosa, and the two diseases may be difficult to separate.[33] BCG[34] is

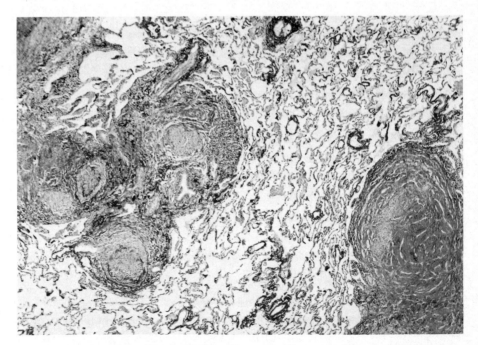

Figure 5–10. Necrotising sarcoidal granulomatosis. Three granulomas on left obliterating pulmonary arteries with fragmentation of elastic lamina. Hyalinised granulomas on the right. Elastic, van Gieson's × 44.

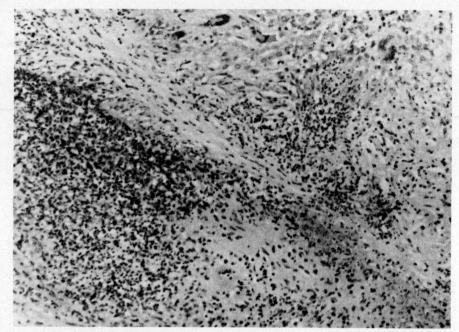

Figure 5–11. Wegener's granulomatosis. Poorly formed granulomas with Wegener's-type atypical giant cells surrounding infarct-like necrotic areas. H & E × 80.

confined to the lungs and is characterised by necrotic eosinophil-rich lesions centred on the bronchi with a surrounding palisade of epithelioid and giant cells. The majority of cases are a form of invasive aspergillosis, and careful search reveals fungal hyphae within the necrotic areas. We are thus reminded that fungi must always be looked for in any doubtful pulmonary granuloma.

LYG,[35] other than the name, has little in common with sarcoidosis. Granulomas are exceptional; the angiocentric lesions consist of primitive lymphocytes and reticulum cells, and around 14 per cent of cases progress to malignant disseminated lymphoma.

SARCOIDOSIS OF THE UPPER RESPIRATORY TRACT

We have observed sarcoidosis of the upper respiratory tract (SURT) in 53 of 818 (6 per cent) patients (Table 5–10). Women were affected twice as often as men (35F:18M). Thirty-seven patients (70 per cent) presented for the first time under the age of 40, and the average age at presentation was 35 (range 11 to 65 years). Caucasians featured most commonly (78 per cent), but there was a significant minority of West Indians (19 per cent), and it was also observed in three Kenyan Asians. These findings are similar to those of the overall series. At the time of presentation 33 (62 per cent) had symptoms of upper respiratory tract sarcoidosis without obvious symptomatic sarcoidosis elsewhere.

Table 5–10. A Comparison of Sarcoidosis of the Upper Respiratory Tract and Sarcoidosis Overall

Feature	Sarcoidosis Overall		SURT	
	Number	*%*	*Number*	*%*
Female	500	61	35	66
Presentation under age 40	604	74	37	70
Caucasian	728	89	41	78
West Indian	81	10	10	19
Intrathoracic	700	88	48	90
Ocular	224	27	16	30
Erythema nodosum	251	31	13	25
Lupus pernio	35	4	15	30
Other skin lesions	117	14	21	40
Bone	31	3	7	11
Lymphadenopathy	225	27	8	15
Splenomegaly	101	12	4	7
Nervous system	77	9	3	6
Parotid	52	6	10	18
Lacrimal gland	22	3	2	4
Upper respiratory tract	53	6	53	100
Systemic corticosteroid therapy	344	42	40	75
Mortality due to				
Sarcoidosis	25	3	3	6
Other causes	23	3	1	2
TOTAL	818	100	53	100

Sites of Involvement

Nasal Mucosa. The nasal mucosa was affected in 36 (69 per cent) patients (Table 5–11). The major symptoms were obstruction, crusting, and discharge. The inferior turbinate and septum were most commonly involved, but occasionally more widespread lesions were noted. Polypoid hypertrophy caused nasal obstruction, and, on examination, the mucosa was usually erythematous and granular (Fig. 5–12).

Laryngeal and Pharyngeal Mucosa. Sarcoidosis of the larynx and pharynx was observed in eight (15 per cent) patients (Figs. 5–13 [see also Color Plate 3] and 5–14). All patients complained of hoarseness, and, in addition to either supra- or subglottic granulomas, there was nasal cavity involvement in all patients. Two patients had marked laryngeal obstruction with stridor due to florid supra- and subglottic granulomas.

Septal Perforation. Nasal septal perforation occurred in three patients. Two had undergone submucosal resection elsewhere to alleviate obstruction, but nasal sarcoidosis remained unrecognised, nasal obstruction being the only presenting symptom. Surgery was complicated by septal perforation in both patients, and one also developed palatal perforation. Both patients progressed to lupus pernio.

Nasal Bone Involvement. In seven patients lateral radiographs of the nasal bones showed abnormalities, and four of these also had bone lesions in the hands or feet or both. Doubtful nasal bone involvement was also seen in another two patients; one had extremity lesions and the other had a

Table 5–11. Sites of Sarcoid Involvement of the Upper Respiratory Tract

Tissue	Number	%
Nasal mucosa	36	69
Laryngeal and pharyngeal mucosa	8	15
Nasal bone	7	13
Sinus	8	15
Parotids	10	18
TOTAL	53	100

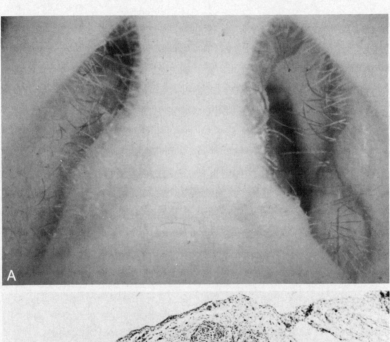

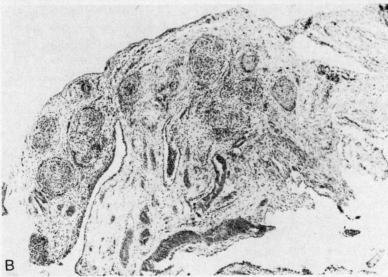

Figure 5–12. A, Sarcoid granulomas in nasal mucosa. B, × 40.

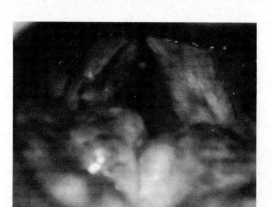

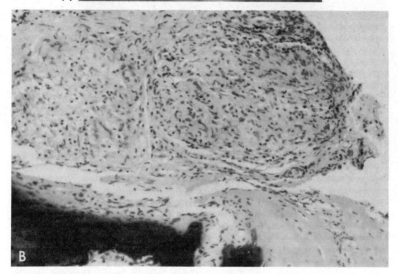

Figure 5–13. *A*, Sarcoid involvement of larynx. *B*, Histology of larynx. × 60.

probable bone lesion in one foot. There was radiographic evidence of surgical intervention of the nose in another two patients.

The normal lateral film of the nasal bones represents the superimposed shadows in both alae. The usual bone texture is compact, often almost structureless, the margins are well defined, and there are linear translucencies due to sutural lines. Sarcoid involvement produces alterations in bone texture of varying degree and extent. The lesions may appear as scattered, punctate areas of porosis or zones of frank destruction. There may be defects due to bone absorption or surgery. In long standing involvement, a wide-meshed trabecular pattern may form. This appears to result from an alteration in the trabecular distribution in response to the presence of granulomas within the bone. In such lesions the suture lines may disappear. No periosteal reaction has been seen.

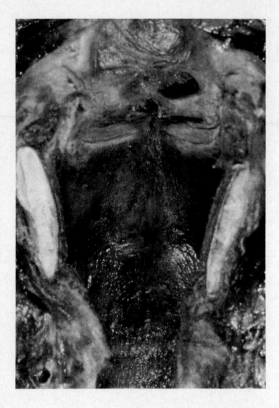

Figure 5–14. SURT fatality. Larynx shows widespread ulceration and granular mucosa. × 3.

Clinical Accompaniment

Multisystem involvement is evident in SURT in much the same way as in the overall series; a comparison highlights their similarities (see Table 5–10).

Intrathoracic involvement was seen in 48 (90 per cent) patients, an incidence similar to that of the overall series. Bilateral hilar lymphadenopathy was predominant, but all three stages of abnormal chest radiographs were noted. Whereas chest x-ray resolution occurred in 52 per cent of patients with sarcoidosis overall, it was only evident in 11 (23 per cent) patients with SURT (Table 5–12).

Ocular involvement occurred in 16 (30 per cent) patients, principally, chronic anterior uveitis in 9, with secondary cataract formation in 2 and glaucoma in 1, all pointing to chronic indolent disease.

Skin lesions were associated with SURT in 49 (92 per cent) patients, comprising plaques or subcutaneous nodules in 21, lupus pernio in 15, and erythema nodosum in 13. Fifteen patients with SURT had lupus pernio, an interesting and common association.[36, 37] There was nasal involvement in all, ranging from a small button-like lesion or a few nodules on the tip of the nose to florid granulomatous lesions involving the skin of the nose and spreading across the cheeks.

Table 5–12. Chest Radiographic Changes in SURT Compared with Sarcoidosis Overall

Radiographical Stage*	SURT		Sarcoidosis Overall	
	Number	*%*	*Number*	*%*
0	5	10	118	14
1	32	60	458	65
2	10	18	150	22
3	6	12	92	13
Total abnormal	48	90	700	86
Resolution	11	23	362	52
Total Series	53	100	818	100

*0 = Normal.
1 = Bilateral hilar lymphadenopathy (BHL).
2 = BHL + pulmonary infiltration.
3 = Pulmonary infiltration.

There may be associated red, swollen, painful digits. It is tempting to postulate spread of the granulomatous process from an initial focus in the nasal mucosa through the nasal bone and then on to the overlying skin. (We have noted a similar association between bone cysts and adjacent soft tissues in the hands and feet.) Septal perforation may accelerate the development of lupus pernio of the overlying skin of the nose.

Parotid gland enlargement was noted in 10 (18 per cent) patients; it was unilateral in 6.

Neurological involvement was evident in two patients with transient unilateral lower motor neuron VII nerve palsies and one with a unilateral XII cranial nerve palsy. Another West Indian female had widespread sarcoid involvement of the brain and hydrocephalus in a CAT scan. She died under anaesthesia for contemplated relief shunt surgery.

Course

Forty (75 per cent) patients needed steroids. Systemic steroids were necessary in 24 (46 per cent); steroids were given with chloroquine in 12 (23 per cent), and topical steroids were sufficient in 4 patients. Intravenous steroids were a matter of urgency in two patients to relieve life-threatening stridor due to laryngeal involvement with airway obstruction; this was just enough to avoid tracheostomy. Four of the 53 patients died, one postoperatively following surgery for peripheral vascular disease, another during cerebral surgery, and two owing to respiratory failure (see Fig. 5–14). The course of the remainder has been chronic fibrotic sarcoidosis in all systems (Table 5–13). Intrathoracic involvement is pulmonary fibrosis leading to respiratory failure. Only 11 (23 per cent) patients achieved a normal chest radiograph compared with 52 per cent overall (see Table 5–12). Likewise, chronic fibrotic disease involves eyes, skin, and bone. Within this setting, it

Table 5–13. Features of SURT Suggestive of a Chronic Progressive Indolent Form

Feature	Acute	Tempo of Sarcoidosis Chronic	SURT
Onset	Abrupt	Insidious	Insidious
Self-limiting	Yes	No	No
Progression	No	Yes	Yes
Complications	No	Yes	Yes
Histology	Exudative	Fibrotic	Fibrotic
Chronic skin lesions	Infrequent	Frequent	Frequent
Chronic uveitis	Infrequent	Frequent	Frequent
Chest x-ray resolution	Frequent	Infrequent	Infrequent

Table 5–14. The Differential Diagnosis of Sarcoid Granulomas of the Upper Respiratory Tract

Feature	Sarcoidosis	Tuberculosis	Leprosy (Tuberculoid)	Wegener's Granulomatosis
Female:male	2:1	1:1	1:1	1:2
Age at onset (years)	30–50	Any	Any	25–55
Race	Any	Asian	Tropical	Any
Clinical involvements				
Skin over nose	Yes (lupus pernio)	Yes (lupus vulgaris)	Yes	No
Skin elsewhere	Yes	No	Yes	Yes
Intrathoracic	Nearly always	Nearly always	No	Frequently
Uveitis	Yes	No	Yes	Yes
Neuropathy	Cranial nerve palsies	Due to isoniazid	Yes	No
Renal failure	Rarely	No	No	Yes
Fever	No	Yes	Yes	Yes
Skin tests				
Tuberculin	Negative	Positive	±	±
Kveim-Siltzbach	Positive	Negative	Negative	Negative
Histology	Granuloma	Granuloma	Granuloma	Granulomatous angiitis
Kidney histology	Nephrocalcinosis	Abscess	Normal	—
Serum angiotensin-converting enzyme level	Elevated	Normal	Normal	Normal
Microbiology	Negative	Mycobacteria	Mycobacteria	Negative
Treatment	Steroids Chloroquine Methotrexate	Rifampicin Isoniazid Ethambutol Pyrazinamide	Dapsone Transfer factor Rifampicin	Steroids Azathioprine Cyclophosphamide

is not surprising that SURT progresses indolently over the years, complicated by nasal bone involvement, septal collapse, and laryngeal obstruction. Also curiously, septal perforation may accelerate the development of lupus pernio of the overlying skin of the nose.

DIAGNOSIS

When a granuloma is found in the upper respiratory tract, the differential diagnosis comprises tuberculosis, extrinsic allergic alveolitis, leprosy, and Wegener's granulomatosis. These conditions must be differentiated, for the natural history, prognosis, and treatment are all very different (Table 5–14).

REFERENCES

1. Battesti JP, Saumon G, Yaleyre D, Amouroux J, Pechnick B, Sandron D, Georges R. Pulmonary sarcoidosis with an alveolar radiographic pattern. Thorax. 37:448, 1982.
2. Harkleread LE, Young RL, Savage PJ, Jenkins DW, London R E. Pulmonary sarcoidosis: Longterm follow-up of the effects of steroid therapy. Chest. 82:84, 1982.
3. Johns CJ, Macgregor IA, Zachary JB, Ball WC. Extended experience in the longterm corticosteroid treatment of pulmonary sarcoidosis. Ann NY Acad Sci. 178:722, 1976.
4. Hunninhake GW, Fulmer JD, Young RC Jr, Gadek JE, Crystal RG. Localisation of the immune response in sarcoidosis. Am Rev Respir Dis. 120:49, 1979.
5. Lawrence EC, Martin RR, Blaese RM, Teague RT, Awe RJ, Wilson RK, Deaton WJ, Bloom K, Greenberg SD, Stevens PM. Increased bronchoalveolar IgG-secretin G cells in interstitial lung diseases. New Engl J Med. 302:1186, 1980.
6. Greening AP. Bronchoalveolar lavage. Br Med J. 284:1896, 1982.
7. Perrin-Fayolle M, Pacheco Y, Harf R, Montagnon B, Biot N. Angiotensin-converting enzyme in bronchoalveolar lavage fluid in pulmonary sarcoidosis. Thorax. 34:790, 1981.
8. Rossi AG, Hunninghake GW, Crystal RG. Evaluation of inflammatory and immune processes in the interstitial lung disorders: Use of bronchoalveolar lavage. In Cumming G, Bonsignore G (eds): Cellular Biology of the Lung. Plenum Press, New York. p 107, 1982.
9. Jones Williams W. Pathology of pulmonary sarcoidosis. Proc Roy Soc Med. 60:986, 1967.
10. Turiaf J, Battesti JP, Marland P, Basset F, Amouroux F. Sarcoidosis involving large pulmonary arteries. In Jones Williams W, Davies BH (eds): Sarcoidosis. Cardiff, Alpha Omega Press. p 3, 1980.
11. Keogh BA, Crystal RG. Alveolitis: the key to interstitial lung disorders. Thorax. 37:1, 1982.
12. Lacronique J, Bernaudin JF, Soler P, Lange F, Kawanami O, Saumon G, Georges R, Basset F. Alveolitis and granulomas: sequential course in pulmonary sarcoidosis. In Chretien J, Marsac J, Saltiel JC (eds): Proc 9th Internat Conf Sarcoidosis. Paris, Pergamon Press. p 36, 1983.
13. Jones Williams W. Beryllium disease—pathology and diagnosis. J Occup Med. 27:93, 1977.
14. Seal RME, Hapke EJ, Thomas GO, Meek JC, Hayes M. The pathology of the acute and chronic stages of Farmer's Lung. Thorax. 23:469, 1968.
15. Izumi T, Kobara Y, Nui S, Tokunga R, Orita Y, Kitano M, Jones Williams W. The first seven cases of chronic beryllium disease in ceramic factory workers in Japan. Ann NY Acad Sci. 278:636, 1976.
16. Sharma OP. Sarcoidosis: unusual pulmonary manifestations. Postgrad Med. 61:67, 1977.
17. Hadfield JW, Page RL, Flower CDR, Stark JE. Localised airways narrowing in sarcoidosis. Thorax. 37:443, 1982.

18. Thunell M, Bjerle P, Stjernberg N. Clinical manifestations and prognosis of bronchostenosis due to sarcoidosis. *In* Chretien J, Marsac J, Saltiel J C (eds): Proc 9th Internat Conf Sarcoidosis. Paris, Pergamon Press. p 306, 1983.

19. Ingram CG, Reid PC, Johnston RN. Exercise testing in pulmonary sarcoidosis. Thorax. 37:129, 1982.

20. Powell E, Renzi G, Macklem PT. Severity and site of airflow obstruction in sarcoidosis. *In* Chretien J, Marsac J, Saltiel JC (eds): Proc 9th Internat Conf Sarcoidosis. Paris, Pergamon Press. p 276, 1983.

21. Bechtel JJ, Starr T, Dantzker DR, Bower JS. Airway hyper-reactivity in patients with sarcoidosis. Am Rev Resp Dis. 124:759, 1981.

22. Bower JS, Dantzker DR. Airway obstruction in sarcoidosis. Am Rev Resp Dis. 115(4):91, 1977.

23. Wollmer P, Rhodes CG, Bowley NB, Hughes JMB. Extravascular lung density in sarcoidosis measured with positron tomography. Proc Br Thorac Assoc and Thoracic Soc. p 238, 1981.

24. Jones Williams W, Williams WR. The value of beryllium lymphocyte transformation tests in chronic beryllium disease and in potentially exposed workers. Thorax 38:41, 1983.

25. Farber HW, Fairman RP, Glaiser FL. Talc granulomatosis: Laboratory findings similar to sarcoidosis. Am Rev Resp Dis. 125:258, 1982.

26. Abraham JL, Brambilla C. Particle size for differentiation between inhalation and injection pulmonary talcosis (abstr). Am Rev Resp Dis. 119:196, 1979.

27. Osband ME, Lipton JM, Lavin P, Levey R, Vawter G, Greenberger JS, et al. Histiocytosis X. Demonstration of abnormal immunity. T-cell histamine H2 receptor deficiency and successful treatment with thymic extract. N Engl J Med. 304:146, 1981.

28. Basset F, Soler P, Wyllie L, Mazin F, Turiaf J. Langerhan's cells and lung interstitium. Ann NY Acad Sci. 278:599, 1976.

29. Basset F, Corrin B, Spencer H, Lacronique J, Roth C, Soler P, Battesti J, Georges R, Chretien J. Pulmonary histiocytosis X. Am Rev Resp Dis. 118:811, 1978.

30. Liebow AA. The J Burns Amberson Lecture. Pulmonary angiitis and granulomatosis. Am Rev Resp Dis. 108:1, 1973.

31. Churg A, Carrington C B, Gupta R. Necrotising sarcoid granulomatosis. Chest. 76:406, 1979.

32. DeRemee RA, McDonald TJ, Weiland LH. Wegener's granulomatosis, polymorphic reticulosis and lymphomatoid granulomatosis: A comparative analysis. *In* Jones Williams W and Davies BH (eds): Sarcoidosis. Cardiff, Alpha and Omega Press. p 738, 1980.

33. Fauci AS, Haynes BF, Katz P. The spectrum of vasculitis, clinical, pathological, immunological and therapeutic considerations. Ann Intern Med. 89:660, 1978.

34. Katzenstein AL, Liebow AA, Friedman PJ. Bronchocentric granulomatosis mucoid impaction and hypersensitivity reactions to fungi. Am Rev Resp Dis. 111:497, 1975.

35. Liebow AA, Carrington CB, Friedman PJ. Lymphomatoid granulomatosis. Human Pathol. 3:457, 1972.

36. Neville E, Mills RGS, Jash DK, McKinnon DM, Carstairs L S. Sarcoidosis of the upper tracts and its association with lupus pernio. Thorax. 31:660, 1976.

37. James DG, Barter S, Jash D, Mackinnon DM, Carstairs LS. Sarcoidosis of the upper respiratory tract. J Laryng and Otol. 96:711, 1982.

38. Neville E, Walker AM, James DG. Prognostic factors predicting the outcome of sarcoidosis: An analysis of 818 patients. Quart J Med. New Series L11, 208:525, 1983.

6

Ocular and Neurosarcoidosis

BACKGROUND

Ocular sarcoidosis has been recognised throughout this century. The earliest descriptions were followed by various ocular syndromes (see Chapter 1), and eventually ocular and neurosarcoidosis became interwoven. In 1937, Waldenström described five patients with bilateral parotid gland enlargement and bilateral uveitis due to sarcoidosis, four of whom were women over 30 years of age.[1] The disease was clearly multisystemic for one or another of these patients had evidence of involvement of the neurological system, lungs, lymph nodes, or skin, as well as fever or hyperglobulinaemia. He drew particular attention to bizarre neurological manifestations that included right facial or hypoglossal nerve palsy and bilateral optic neuritis and at the same time indicated meningeal involvement with cerebrospinal fluid pleocytosis. A decade later, Colover, in 1948, uncovered papilloedema in 16 of 118 cases of neurosarcoidosis.[2] The cerebrospinal fluid was abnormal in 23 of these patients.

Ocular sarcoidosis, including papilloedema, is now well recognised in Britain[3, 4] and also worldwide. In a worldwide survey of sarcoidosis, there was a variable incidence of ocular disease[5] (Table 6–1).

Since ocular sarcoidosis is but one feature of a systemic disorder, it is important to be aware of its many facets (Fig. 6–1), and the ophthalmologist is well advised to follow the full investigative routine recommended (see Chapter 4, p. 44).

OCULAR LESIONS

Uveitis occurs in about one-fourth of patients with sarcoidosis; conversely, sarcoidosis is the cause in a mere 5 per cent of patients with uveitis. In our series 224 patients (27 per cent) had ocular involvement. They were most frequent in the 20- to 40-year age group, and twice as often they were females. The most common lesion was anterior uveitis (in 66 per cent), followed by posterior uveitis in 14 per cent, anterior and posterior uveitis in 13 per cent, conjunctival lesions in 19 per cent, and scleral plaques in 2 per cent of patients (Fig. 6–2). The relative infrequency of posterior uveitis is artificial, since it is difficult to detect in the presence of acute inflammation of the anterior segment of the eye. Now that anterior uveitis is rapidly being

Table 6–1. Incidence of Ocular Sarcoidosis and Neurosarcoidosis in a Worldwide Survey of 3,676 Patients in 11 Cities

City	Number of Patients	Ocular Sarcoidosis		Neurosarcoidosis	
		No.	%	No.	%
London	537	147	27	38	7
New York	311	62	20	13	4
Paris	350	37	11	16	4
Los Angeles	150	17	11	3	2
Tokyo	282	91	32	11	4
Reading	425	69	16	39	9
Lisbon	89	5	6	4	4
Edinburgh	502	53	11	15	3
Novi Sad	285	43	15	4	1.4
Naples	624	0	0	0	0
Geneva	121	15	12	1	1
Total	3,676	539	15	144	4

*Data from James DG, Neville E, Siltzbach LE, et al.: A world-wide review of sarcoidosis. Ann NY Acad Sci. 278:321, 1976.

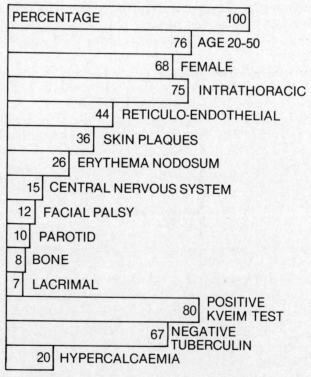

Figure 6–1. Clinical and other associations of ocular sarcoidosis in our series of 224 patients.

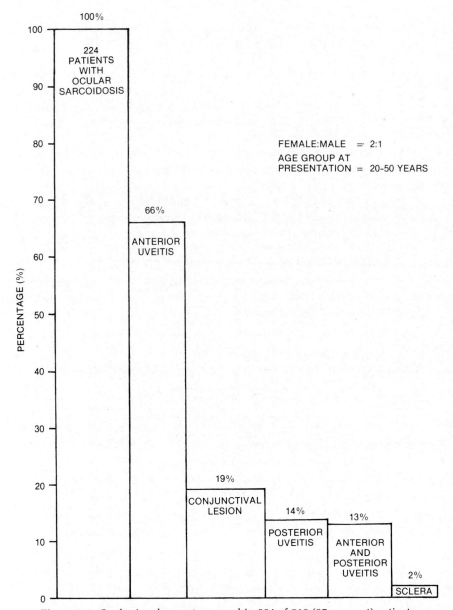

Figure 6–2. Ocular involvement occurred in 224 of 818 (27 per cent) patients.

brought under control by corticosteroids, it is possible to examine the fundus oculi at a much earlier stage when sarcoid lesions are still present. Consequently, posterior uveitis is less likely to be overlooked in the future.

ANTERIOR UVEITIS

Anterior uveitis can be subdivided into acute or chronic iridocyclitis, depending on the onset, course, duration, and clinical associations (Table 6–2, Fig. 6–3). Acute sarcoid iridocyclitis (Fig. 6–4; see also color plate 4) has an abrupt onset, appears most often in women in the 20- to 30-year age group, and is sometimes associated with erythema nodosum and bilateral hilar lymphadenopathy. It responds well to local corticosteroid therapy, and the whole course usually subsides uneventfully in a matter of weeks or months.

By way of contrast, chronic sarcoid iridocyclitis has an insidious onset in an older age group. Ocular fibrosis leads to secondary glaucoma and cataract formation, so the prolonged course is often measured in terms of years or a lifetime. Lesions in other systems—lupus pernio, bone cysts, and pulmonary fibrosis—also reflect irreversible tissue fibrosis. Steroids may provide some symptomatic relief, but their long-term use is undesirable, and chloroquine, despite its ocular toxicity, or methotrexate may be considered as alternative antifibrotic treatments.

Table 6–2. Differences Between Acute and Chronic Iridocyclitis Due to Sarcoidosis

Feature	Acute	Chronic
Onset	Abrupt	Insidious
Decade of onset (years)	20–35	35–50
Course	Transient	Persistent
Signs	Ciliary congestion Turbid aqueous Keratic precipitates	Fatty nodules Synechiae
Sequelae	Rare	Lens opacities Glaucoma Cataract Blindness
Chest radiograph	Hilar adenopathy	Pulmonary fibrosis
Skin lesions	Erythema nodosum	Lupus pernio
Bone cysts	No	Yes
Response to corticosteroids	Good	Poor
Alternative treatment	Oxyphenbutazone Indomethacin	Chloroquine Methotrexate

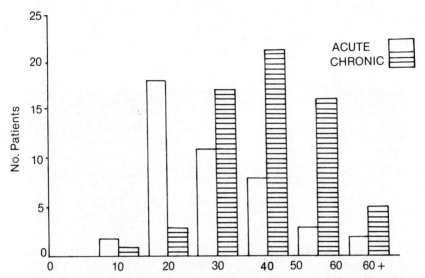

Figure 6–3. Age distribution in acute versus chronic sarcoid uveitis. Acute uveitis starts in an earlier age group and rarely presents in those over 50. Chronic uveitis presents insidiously and is frequent in the 40- to 60-year age group.

POSTERIOR UVEITIS

There are many descriptive reports of lesions of the posterior segment, including choroidoretinitis,[6-8] papilloedema,[3] periphlebitis retinae,[9] and retinal haemorrhage.[10, 11]

A recent review of the fundus changes in 36 patients with ocular sarcoidosis indicates that all had a vitreous cellular infiltrate; periphlebitis was present in three-quarters of patients, followed in order of frequency by disc oedema and changes in the subretinal pigment epithelium. The disease has a low visual morbidity unless neovascularisation develops.[12]

Choroidal nodules are usually scattered discrete off-white waxy exudates, sometimes causing retinal venous constriction and periphlebitis (Fig. 6–5). These lesions were first described by Walsh.[13] In 1949, Franceschetti and Babel used the term *choroido-retinitis "en tache de bougie"* to describe this appearance.[14] Peripheral choroiditis is symptomless. Involvement of the macula causes blurring and loss of vision (Fig. 6–6). Fundal lesions are painless, but an associated anterior lesion may cause pain. The more severe the posterior lesion, the greater the probability that it will be associated with some anterior manifestation of the disease. Fluorescein angiography has brought a new dimension to the assessment of sarcoid uveitis, for leakage of dye displays with clarity the retinal vasculitis (Fig. 6–7).

There is a close relationship between granuloma formation and blood vessels; this is particularly evident in the central nervous system in the walls of veins and capillaries, producing granulomatous periphlebitis. This is shown most elegantly by venous leakage with fluorescein angiography in retinal sarcoidosis.

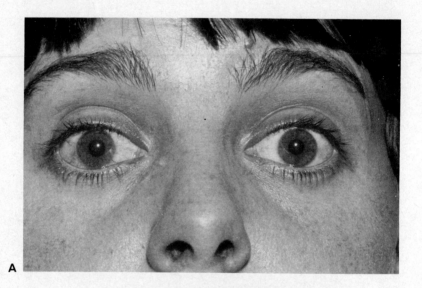

A

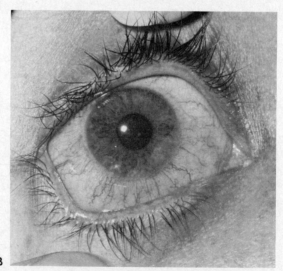

B

Figure 6–4. *A* and *B*, Acute iritis.

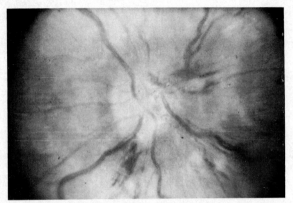

Figure 6–5. Retinal sarcoidosis.

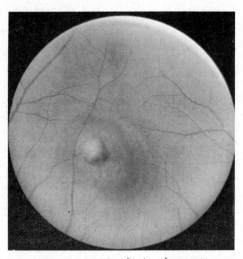

Figure 6–6. Macular involvement.

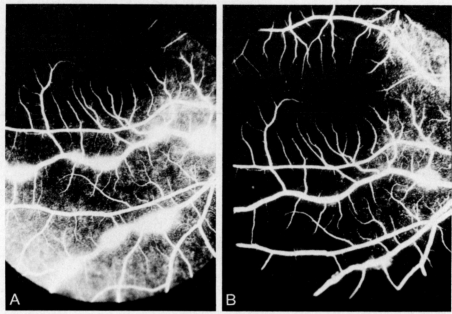

Figure 6–7. Fluorescein angiogram of retinal vasculitis due to sarcoidosis. *A*, Before treatment. *B*, Three weeks after oral prednisolone treatment there is considerably less leakage of dye.

PAPILLOEDEMA

Papilloedema (Fig. 6–8) is more frequent in women than in men and is commonly associated with facial palsy and also with pain and hyperalgesia of bizarre distribution on the trunk mimicking pleurisy, appendicitis, or spinal arthritis.[15, 16] One of our patients so afflicted endeavoured to claim compensation for a minor chest injury, which he felt was the cause of his condition.[17] The cerebrospinal fluid and pressure may be normal; in one-half of patients there may be increased protein and cells.

In patients with papilloedema, the diagnosis of neurological sarcoidosis should be entertained when it develops rapidly in adults, particularly women, and also especially if there is facial weakness or other cranial nerve palsies or unusual sensory symptoms over the trunk.

In our reported series of patients with papilloedema due to sarcoidosis, evidence of multisystem involvement, histological evidence of sarcoid tissue, the positive Kveim-Siltzbach test, a gratifying response to corticosteroids, and a subsequent benign course all served to differentiate neurosarcoidosis from the alternative diagnosis of a cerebral tumour.[3] We may now add the value of the CAT scan, which has assumed paramount importance in the differential diagnosis.

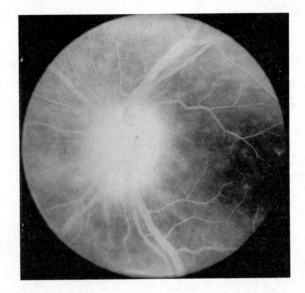

Figure 6–8. Papilloedema.

CONJUNCTIVAL INVOLVEMENT

Phlyctenular, or non-specific, conjunctivitis is more commonly bilateral than unilateral and often coincides with erythema nodosum and bilateral hilar lymphadenopathy as a manifestation of acute, transient sarcoidosis. We have observed it in 28 patients, and granulomas were obtained by biopsy from obvious phlyctenules when they were readily seen.

Conjunctival follicles (Fig. 6–9) have been noted in only nine patients in our series. Granulomas were readily obtained on biopsy of these follicles, which appear as nodular collections in the conjunctival folds of the lower eyelids.

Keratoconjunctivitis sicca is bilateral in women nearing menopause. It is a manifestation of chronic fibrotic sarcoidosis. The dry eyes show corneal staining and degenerative changes, but corneal ulceration is not a feature of sarcoidosis. It is accompanied by other chronic persistent features including enlarged lacrimal and parotid glands, splenomegaly, lymphadenopathy, and pulmonary fibrosis.

Scleritis is a manifestation of acute sarcoidosis, associated with erythema nodosum and bilateral hilar lymphadenopathy and suggesting that it is one component of a circulating immune complex disorder.

Blind Conjunctival Biopsy

Sarcoid granulomas are readily obtained from obvious conjunctival follicles and phlyctenules, but blind biopsy of the conjunctiva is unrewarding.

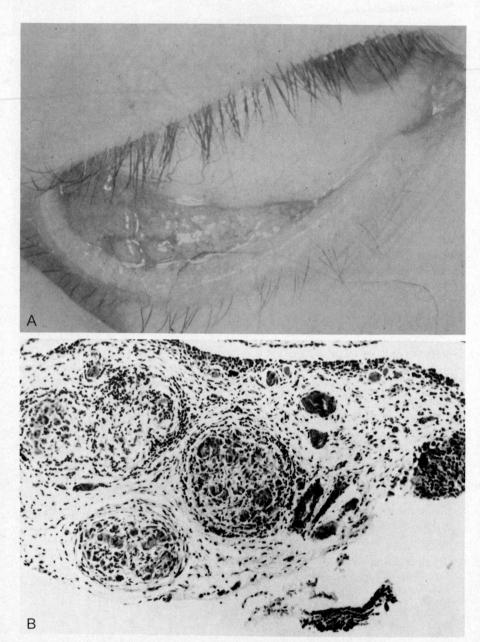

Figure 6–9. *A,* Conjunctival follicles. *B,* Conjunctival biopsy showing three discrete granulomas. H & E × 80.

The vast majority of patients with uveitis have a normal conjunctiva. Unravelling the riddle of uveitis, whether due to sarcoidoss or its many other causes, primarily involves obtaining diagnostic histology; blind biopsy of the normal-looking conjunctiva is rarely helpful (see Chapter 3).

OCULAR SYNDROMES

The literature abounds with descriptive syndromes, some of them eponymous and all of them emphasising the multisystem character of sarcoidosis (Fig. 6–10).

Heerfordt's Syndrome[18]

This could equally well have been termed Waldenström's syndrome.[1] It is characterised by uveitis and parotid gland enlargement, runs a chronic and usually febrile course, and is frequently complicated by cranial nerve palsies, especially of the VII cranial nerve. Other components include bizarre

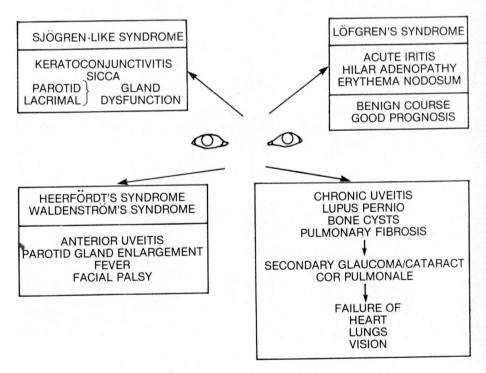

Figure 6–10. Clinical syndromes of ocular sarcoidosis.

neurological manifestations, lethargy, hyperalgesia, meningism, papilloedema, and cerebrospinal fluid pleocytosis.

In our series of 818 patients with sarcoidosis (see Table 4–1) we observed parotid gland enlargement in 52 (6 per cent) and uveitis in 224 (27 per cent). Conversely, in a series of 147 patients with ocular sarcoidosis, parotid gland enlargement occurred in 10 per cent and facial palsy in 12 per cent.[19]

Löfgren's Syndrome[20]

The late Sven Löfgren of Stockholm (see p. 8) delineated the association of erythema nodosum and bilateral hilar lymphadenopathy due to sarcoidosis. Uveitis occurred in 13 of 212 patients (6 per cent), with roughly the same incidence in cases with and without erythema nodosum. Eight of the 13 patients with uveitis had concurrent parotitis.[20] Löfgren's syndrome is associated with acute iritis. The syndrome is self-limiting and carries a good prognosis with ultimate complete resolution of sarcoidosis.

Sjögren's-like Syndrome

Keratoconjunctivitis sicca with or without parotid and lacrimal gland involvement mimics Sjögren's syndrome with its distressing symptoms of dry eyes and dry mouth (Fig. 6–11), but there is no arthritis, which is such a prominent feature of Sjögren's syndrome.

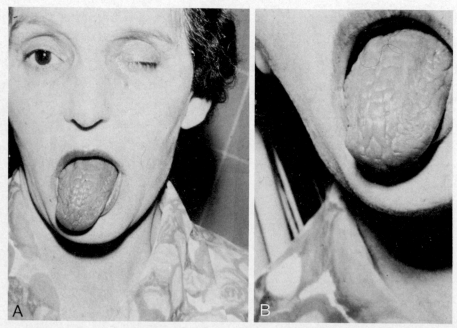

Figure 6–11. *A* and *B*, Sjögren's-like syndrome with dry eyes and dry tongue, and protective tarsorrhaphy to left eye.

Chronic Uveitis

Chronic fibrotic sarcoidosis may present insidiously with longstanding subacute or chronic uveitis, lupus pernio, bone cysts, and pulmonary fibrosis (Fig. 6–12). Irreversible fibrosis has occurred in all systems, so ultimate resolution is unlikely to occur. Systemic steroids may provide symptomatic relief but do not quell the underlying fibrosis.

NEUROSARCOIDOSIS

We have observed neurosarcoidosis in 77 of our 818 patients (9 per cent) and in 4 per cent of patients worldwide (see Table 4–1). In our initial detailed analysis in London, neurosarcoidosis occurred in 38 of 537 patients (7 per cent) (Table 6–3), with features and distribution similar to those of other series.[21]

Facial palsy was the most frequent neurological presentation, occurring in 25 patients either alone or with other cranial nerve palsies (in 4) or with papilloedema (in 3) (Fig. 6–13). It occurred equally often unilaterally, either right or left in nine, and bilaterally, in seven patients. Resolution was complete in 80 per cent of this group.

Papilloedema was noted in seven patients. It is accompanied by haemorrhages, exudates, vasculitis, anterior uveitis, facial weakness, and bizarre paraesthesiae of the trunk and involvement of other systems.

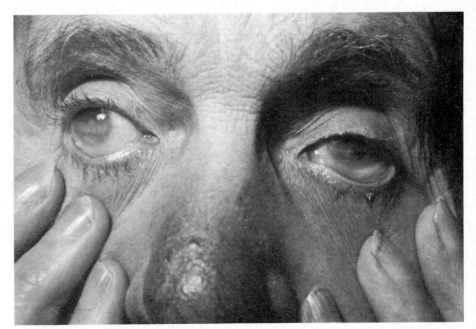

Figure 6–12. Chronic uveitis leading to blindness. The patient also has lupus pernio involving the nose and nasal mucosa.

Table 6–3. Features of Neurosarcoidosis in 38 of 537 Patients in London Series

	Patients	
Feature	*Number*	*%*
Females	21	55
Age 21–30 years	13 ⎫	
31–40	9 ⎬	81
41–50	9 ⎭	
51–60	5	14
> 60	2	5
Facial nerve palsy	25	66
Other cranial nerve palsies	12	31
Papilloedema	7	18
Peripheral neuritis	7	18
CSF pressure/protein raised	9	24
Epilepsy	2	5
Intracranial mass	1	2
Meningitis	1	2
Cerebellar ataxia	1	2
Intrathoracic involvement	31	82
Eye lesions	22	60
Skin lesions	11	30
Peripheral lymphadenopathy	10	26
Splenomegaly	4	10
Enlarged lacrimals	2	5
Bone cysts	1	2
Enlarged parotids	6	16
Positive Kveim test	22/29	76
Negative tuberculin test	18/30	60
Raised serum globulins	10/30	33
Hypercalcaemia	11/36	30
Total	38/537	7

Other manifestations include peripheral neuropathy, meningitis, space-occupying brain lesions, epilepsy, cerebellar ataxia, hypopituitarism, and diabetes insipidus. Most patients are 20 to 50 years of age, and there is evidence of intrathoracic involvement in 82 per cent, ocular disease in 58 per cent, and splenomegaly in 10 per cent. Neurosarcoidosis carries a mortality of 10 per cent, which is more than twice the overall mortality of sarcoidosis. Resolution of neurosarcoidosis is more likely to occur in younger patients after an explosive onset. The response to corticosteroid therapy is better in those with accompanying erythema nodosum than in those with chronic skin lesions, in those with acute rather than chronic uveitis, and in those with hilar adenopathy rather than old diffuse pulmonary infiltration.

Meningitis may be acute or chronic. The course and prognosis depend on the presentation. An acute and sudden onset is similar to that of any other meningitis that enters into the differential diagnosis. Once the diagnosis has been made, steroid therapy is dramatic and effective. By way of contrast, insidious-onset, low-grade meningitis grumbles along relentlessly. There may be an encouraging initial response to steroids, but relapses occur

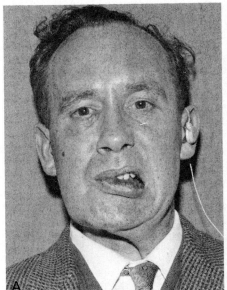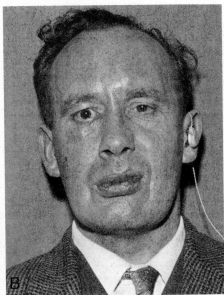

Figure 6–13. Facial palsy and deafness.

when steroids are discontinued or the dose is reduced below a critical level. This state of affairs may continue for up to five years.

Space-occupying nodular cerebral lesions are now being recognised with increased frequency as a result of CAT scanning (Fig. 6–14). Symptoms and signs mimic those of cerebral tumour. Space-occupying nodular cerebral lesions constitute a chronic form of the disease and are most difficult to treat because symptoms persist despite steroids or a combination of steroids and azathioprine. If these drugs fail, then radiotherapy should be considered. The presence of internal hydrocephalus also carries a gloomy prognosis, for it is unrelieved by medical means and surgery carries a considerable operative risk.

Polyneuropathy is a rare neurological manifestation of sarcoidosis. The patient complains of paraesthesia and weakness in the limbs. The chest x-ray may be normal, but lung function tests reveal severe impairment of ventilation with mild restrictive and diffusion capacity defects. Sural nerve biopsy reveals multiple sarcoid granulomas in the epineural spaces, periangiitis, panangiitis, and axonal degeneration.

Examination of the *spinal fluid* is disappointingly unhelpful in neurosarcoidosis. We note raised pressure and elevated protein levels in one-half of patients in which it is performed, but there is an equal number of patients in which it is normal despite neurological changes. It is of limited diagnostic value.

Autopsy studies have shown that granulomas are most abundant over the base of the brain,[22] with involvement of both veins and arteries (Fig. 6–15). Intracerebral and nerve lesions may consist of granulomatous nodules

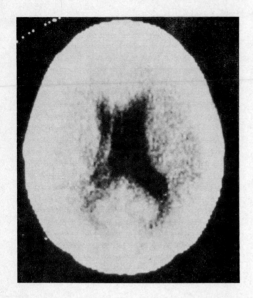

Figure 6–14. CAT scan reveals hydro-cephalus due to sarcoidosis.

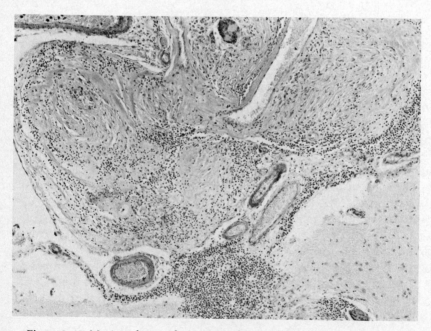

Figure 6–15. Meningeal sarcoidosis. Note relation to blood vessels. H & E × 50.

(Fig. 6–16), isolated granulomas, or scars in which Schaumann's bodies may be present.[23] The histological diagnosis depends on excluding known cases of neurogranulomas (Fig. 6–17) and evidence of multisystem diseases.

Hypothalamic Manifestations of Sarcoidosis

Neural involvement at the base of the brain is uncommon in sarcoidosis but well described, whereas hypothalamic-pituitary dysfunction is very rare.

Hyperprolactinaemia, although rare, is well-recognised. Turkington and MacIndoe observed it in 11 patients (3 men, 8 women) with sarcoidosis.[24] In three patients with the galactorrhoea-amenorrhoea syndrome, treatment with L-dopa suppressed prolactin secretion with cessation of galactorrhoea, resumption of menses, and increased gonadotrophin secretion. A subsequent autopsy in one male showed sarcoid granulomas in the hypothalamic nuclei.

Caro and associates encountered five cases of hyperprolactinaemia in 300 women with sarcoidosis.[25] Pituitary function studies were normal except for elevated serum prolactin levels, which responded normally to L-dopa and thyrotropin-releasing hormone (TRH) but not to chlorpromazine. The response to standard stimulation tests for growth and luteinizing hormone were measured in 7 patients with cerebral sarcoidosis, 15 patients with no evidence of cerebral involvement, and 15 normal subjects. Impaired growth

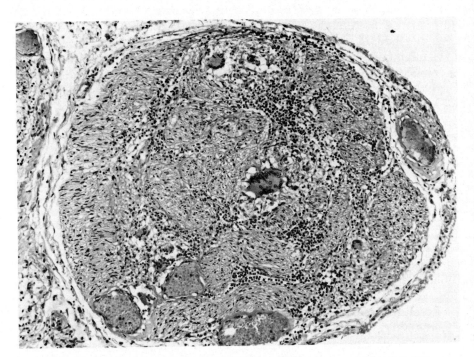

Figure 6–16. Sarcoid granulomas involving posterior nerve root. H & E × 100.

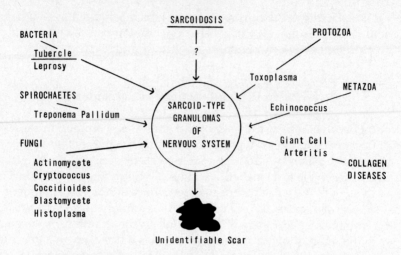

Figure 6–17. Differential histological diagnosis of sarcoid-type granulomas of the nervous system.

and luteinizing hormone responses occurred in six of the seven patients with cerebral sarcoidosis but in none of the others. Malarkey and Kataria noted hyperprolactinaemia in only 1 of 26 patients.[26]

Serum prolactin levels were measured in 50 of our female sarcoidosis patients, 20 with acute and 30 with chronic disease. None of the patients had evidence of cerebral involvement. One patient with an unsuspected pregnancy had an elevated prolactin level. Repeat estimations were normal in five other patients who had borderline elevated prolactin levels but without the galactorrhoea-amenorrhoea syndrome. It seems doubtful whether an isolated measurement of prolactin provides helpful information about cerebral sarcoidosis.

Hypothalamic hypothyroidism also might be expected to occur and Campbell and colleagues have recently described two cases in which this condition was present.[27]

Prognosis

Neurosarcoidosis, like myocardial sarcoidosis, has a poor prognosis with increased morbidity and mortality. In our series, 4 of 38 patients (10 per cent) died as a direct result of sarcoidosis. Diabetes insipidus, epilepsy, and papilloedema are residual defects. Facial palsy subsided completely in four-fifths, and in the remainder there was slight residual facial weakness.

Resolution of neurosarcoidosis is more likely to occur in younger patients whose sarcoidosis has an abrupt onset and a short history; in those with erythema nodosum rather than chronic skin lesions; in those with acute rather than chronic uveitis; and in those with hilar adenopathy rather than old diffuse pulmonary infiltration.

Table 6–4. Chest X-Ray Changes at Presentation and Incidence of
Resolution in 38 Patients with Neurosarcoidosis

Intrathoracic Stage	Patients at Presentation		Resolution	
	No.	*%*	*No.*	*%*
0	7	18	—	—
1	14	37	9	64
2	10	27	4	40
3	7	18	2	29
Total	38	100	15	39

Helpful Investigations

Chest radiography reveals abnormalities in four-fifths of patients (Table 6–4). The course of the chest x-ray changes mirrors changes of the nervous system. Resolving hilar and lung changes are associated with acute meningitis and facial nerve palsy; irreversible pulmonary fibrosis is associated with unchanging space-occupying brain lesions.

CAT scanning must be done early, because it provides much useful information and saves the patient from many unpleasant invasive techniques. Placing this technique second on the list of helpful investigations is realistic, but it may be regarded as a counsel of perfection beyond the reach of Third World countries.

REFERENCES

1. Waldenström J. Some observations of uveoparotitis and allied conditions with special reference to the symptoms from the nervous system. Acta Med Scand. 91:53, 1937.
2. Colover J. Sarcoidosis of the nervous system. Brain. 71:451, 1948.
3. James DG, Zatouroff MA, Trowell J, Rose FC. Papilloedema in sarcoidosis. Br J Ophthal. 51:526, 1967.
4. James DG, Neville E, Langley DA. Ocular sarcoidosis. Trans Ophthalmol Soc (UK). 96:133, 1976.
5. James DG, Neville E, Siltzbach LE, et al. A world-wide review of sarcoidosis. Ann NY Acad Sci. 278:321, 1976.
6. Ainslie D, James DG. Sarcoidosis with ocular involvement. Arch Middlesex Hosp. 3:71, 1953.
7. Gould H, Kaufman HE. Sarcoid of the fundus. Arch Ophthalmol. 65:453, 1961.
8. James DG. The diagnosis and treatment of ocular sarcoidosis. Acta Med Scand Suppl. 425:203, 1964.
9. Ainslie D, James DG. Ocular sarcoidosis. Br Med J. 1:954, 1956.
10. Dow DS. Ocular sarcoidosis. Report of a case characterized by vitreous and retinal hemorrhage, extensive phlebitis, anterior uveitis and secondary glaucoma and with extensive multiple and system involvement. Am J Ophthalmol. 59:93, 1965.
11. Quock GP, Donohoe, RF. Flame shaped retinal haemorrhages in sarcoidosis. J Am Med Assoc. 202:239, 1967.

12. Spalton DJ, Sanders MD. Fundus changes in histologically confirmed sarcoidosis. Br J Ophthal. 65:348, 1981.
13. Walsh FE. Ocular importance of sarcoid. Arch Ophthalmol (Chicago). 21:421, 1939.
14. Franceschetti A, Babel J. La chorionretinite en "tac es de bougie" manifestation de la maladie Besnier-Boeck. Ophthalmologica. 118:701, 1949.
15. Mathews WB. Sarcoidosis of the nervous system. J Neurol Neurosurg Psychiat. 28:23, 1965.
16. Silverstein A, Feuer MM, Siltzbach LE. Neurologic sarcoidosis. Arch Neurol (Chicago). 12:1, 1965.
17. James DG, Sharma OP. Neurological complications of sarcoidosis. Proc Roy Soc Med. 60:1169, 1967.
18. Heerfordt CF. Ueber ein Febris uveo-parotidea sub chronica an der Glandula parotis unter der Uvea des Auges lokalisiert und haufig mit Paresen-cerebrospinaler Nerven kompliziert. Albrecht V Graefes Arch Ophthal. 70:254, 1909.
19. Greenberg G, Anderson R, Sharpstone P, James DG. Enlargement of parotid gland due to sarcoidosis. Br Med J. 2:861, 1964.
20. Löfgren S. Erythema nodosum, studies on aetiology and pathogenesis in 185 adult cases. Acta Med Scand. 124:Suppl 174, 1946.
21. Herring Ab, Urich H. Sarcoidosis of the central nervous system. J Neurol Sci. 9:405, 1969.
22. Matsushita M, Harada K, Matsui Y, Mikami R. Sarcoidosis of the central nervous system. *In* Jones Williams W, Davies BH (eds): Sarcoidosis. Cardiff, Alpha and Omega Press. p. 9, 1980.
23. Jones Williams W. The identification of sarcoid granulomas in the nervous system. Proc Roy Soc Med. 60:38, 1967.
24. Turkington RW, MacIndoe JH. Hyperprolactinaemia in sarcoidosis. Ann Intern Med. 76:545, 1972.
25. Caro JF, Glennon JA, Israel HL. Neuroendocrine studies in sarcoidosis. *In* Jones Williams W, Davies BH (eds): Sarcoidosis. Cardiff, Alpha and Omega Press. p. 587, 1980.
26. Malarkey WB, Kataria YP. Sarcoidosis and hyperprolactinaemia. Ann Intern Med. 81:116, 1974.
27. Campbell IW, Short AIK, Douglas AC. Hypothalamic manifestations of sarcoidosis, with particular reference to hypothalamic hypothyroidism. *In* Jones Williams W, Davies BH (eds): Sarcoidosis. Cardiff, Alpha and Omega Press. p. 579, 1980.

7

The Skin

Skin involvement is common and is frequently associated with erythema nodosum. We have observed and kept under continuous supervision a large series of patients with involvement of the skin by erythema nodosum (251), plaques (76), maculo-papular eruptions (48), sarcoid scars (42), and lupus pernio (35) (Table 7–1).[1-3]

In the worldwide series, erythema nodosum was a mode of presentation of sarcoidosis in 640 of 3,676 (17 per cent) patients; other skin lesions were noted in 324 (9 per cent) (Table 7–2).[4] Some of these skin lesions have a peculiar and interesting association with other systems. In the world review, cutaneous sarcoidosis was associated with intrathoracic involvement in 87 per cent of patients, peripheral lymphadenopathy in 22 per cent, ocular disease in 15 per cent, parotid enlargement or neurosarcoidosis in 4 per cent, and bone involvement in 3 per cent.

ERYTHEMA NODOSUM

We have observed erythema nodosum (Fig. 7–1) due to sarcoidosis in 251 patients. It may be present in any season but is predominant in the spring (Fig. 7–2). The characteristic red, hot, tender, shining, symmetrical lesions on the shins are frequently seen on the calves, knees, and buttocks and sometimes on the arms as well. Some constitutional disturbance is usual at the onset, with swinging fever, even up to 105° F for the first few days, accompanied by troublesome polyarthralgia. The development of the skin

Table 7–1. Skin manifestations in a series of 818 patients with histologically confirmed sarcoidosis*

Skin Lesion	Number	%
Erythema nodosum	251	34
Other lesions	147	18
Plaques	76	9
Maculo-papular rash	48	6
Sarcoid scars	42	5
Lupus pernio	35	4

*There were 147 skin lesions other than erythema nodosum.

Table 7–2. Incidence of involvement of sarcoidosis of the skin in a series of 3,676 patients in 11 cities*

City	Investigators	Patients			Erythema Nodosum		Other Skin Lesions	
		No.	% Female	% Under Age 40 at Presentation	No.	%	No.	%
London	D G James E Neville	537	56	67	167	31	135	25
New York	L E Siltzbach	311	68	71	33	11	59	19
Paris	J Turiaf J P Battesti	350	45	72	22	7	39	12
Los Angeles	O P Sharma	150	67	69	14	9	31	27
Tokyo	Y Hosoda R Mikami M Odaka	282	47	74	10	4	33	12
Reading	A Karlish	425	62	64	134	32	55	13
Lisbon	T G Villar	89	44	72	11	12	16	18
Edinburgh	A C Douglas W Middleton	502	64	72	167	33	34	7
Novi Sad	B Djuric	285	60	37	31	11	12	4
Naples	A Blasi D Olivieri	624	53	77	38	6	3	0.4
Geneva	D Press	121	47	79	13	11	7	6
Total		3,676	57	68	640	17	424	11

*Data from James DG, Neville E, Siltzbach LE, et al. A worldwide review of sarcoidosis. Ann NY Acad Sci. 278:321, 1976.

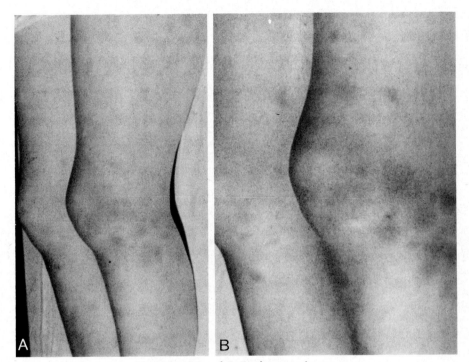

Figure 7–1. *A* and *B,* Erythema nodosum.

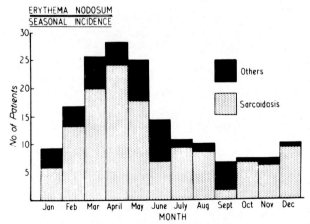

Figure 7–2. Erythema nodosum is predominant in the springtime.

lesions from the onset through the play of colours to the end of bruising occupies 3 weeks but ranges from 1 to 20 weeks (see Fig. 4–2).

Recurrences occur in 10 per cent, usually within 3 months but rarely up to 12 months later. Polyarthralgia, usually of the ankles and knees but sometimes generalised, is experienced by over one-half of patients; it most commonly occurs during the fortnight preceding or following the onset of erythema nodosum, but it may occur up to six weeks before appearance of the eruption. Polyarthralgia preceding erythema nodosum may be indistinguishable from acute rheumatism, for the distribution of flitting pains, fever, sweating, and a grossly elevated sedimentation rate are common to both. The absence of a cardiac murmur and normal electrocardiographical findings are helpful differentiating points, and the subsequent appearance of erythema nodosum, bilateral hilar lymphadenopathy, and a positive Kveim-Siltzbach test are decisive. Accompanying bilateral hilar lymphadenopathy subsided in most patients within one year or so (see Fig. 4–3).

During the years 1960 to 1974, various large series have defined certain causes. Analysis of the pooled data of 1,043 patients in various countries indicates that sarcoidosis is recognised as a cause in about one-third and streptococcal infections in one-fifth of patients; the cause is unknown in about one-quarter of patients (Table 7–3, Fig. 7–3).

Irrespective of the precipitating cause, the ultimate development of polyarthralgia and erythema nodosum depends on racial or constitutional predisposition and hormonal and even geographical factors. It is common in women of the childbearing years and in association with pregnancy and lactation. It is particularly evident among Irish women in London, Puerto Rican women in New York, and Martinique women in Paris. It is a presentation of histoplasmosis in Ohio, coccidioidomycosis in California, leprosy in Africa, and tuberculosis in India. In Europe polyarthralgia and erythema nodosum are common presentations of sarcoidosis. Oral contraceptives may precipitate its development. In his pioneer studies, Löfgren emphasised this interplay of factors, particularly with pelvic inflammation, pregnancy and lactation, gallbladder disease, and streptococcal infection.[5]

Erythema nodosum pinpoints the onset of sarcoidosis in 600 of 3,676 (10 per cent) patients in the worldwide sarcoidosis survey. The distribution was interestingly uneven, for it occurred in one-third of each of the three British series (London, Edinburgh, and Reading) but was less evident elsewhere (Fig. 7–4). It was never a presenting feature of sarcoidosis in Tokyo.[4]

LUPUS PERNIO

Lupus pernio (Fig. 7–5), or purple lupus, was first described by Ernest Besnier in 1889 as a chronic, persistent, violaceous skin lesion with a predilection for the nose, cheeks, and ears.[6] It ranges from a few small

Table 7–3. Conditions Associated With Erythema Nodosum

Associated Disease	Age	Clinical Features	X-Ray	Skin Test	Laboratory Confirmation
Sarcoidosis	20–40, rare below 20	Female preponderance Lymphadenopathy Uveitis or conjunctivitis	Bilateral hilar adenopathy +/– pulmonary infiltration	Kveim-Siltzbach test positive in 94% Tuberculin test negative in 56%	Histology of inflamed scar tissue
Streptococcal infection	Any	Preceding upper respiratory tract infection	—	—	β haemolytic streptococcus in throat Raised anti-streptolysin titre
Tuberculosis	Under 20	Close contact with tuberculosis Primary complex	Unilateral hilar adenopathy Ghon focus	Tuberculin conversion to high degree of positivity	Isolation of *Mycobacterium tuberculosis*
Drugs	Any	Transfer factor Sulphonamides Oral contraceptives Sulphones, penicillin	—	—	Recurs when rechallenged with drug
Histoplasmosis	Any	From Ohio Respiratory symptoms Lymphadenopathy	Miliary mottling	Histoplasmin	CFT Fungal hyphae in sputum or lung biopsy
Coccidioidomycosis	Any	From California Respiratory symptoms Flu-like illness	Miliary mottling Hilar glands or cavitation	Coccidioidin	CFT Fungus in sputum or lung biopsy
Leprosy (lepromatous)	Any	From "Tropics" Symmetrical nodular rash Iridocyclitis Patchy sensory loss	Normal	—	Isolate *M. leprae*: skin or nerve biopsy
Ulcerative colitis	15–40	Diarrhoea	Barium enema	—	Rectal biopsy
Crohn's disease	15–40	Abdominal pain Fever Fistulae	Barium follow through, barium enema	Depression of delayed-type hypersensitivity	Intestinal biopsy
Yersinia infection	Any	Particularly France and Scandinavia Abdominal pain, diarrhoea	Normal chest radiograph and barium studies	—	Stool culture: *Y. enterocolitica* Raised agglutinin titres
Pregnancy	15–40	First trimester	—	—	Recurs with next pregnancy
Behçet's disease	15–40	Orogenital ulceration Thrombophlebitis Ocular inflammation Pyoderma	—	Dermatographia Histamine wheal	—

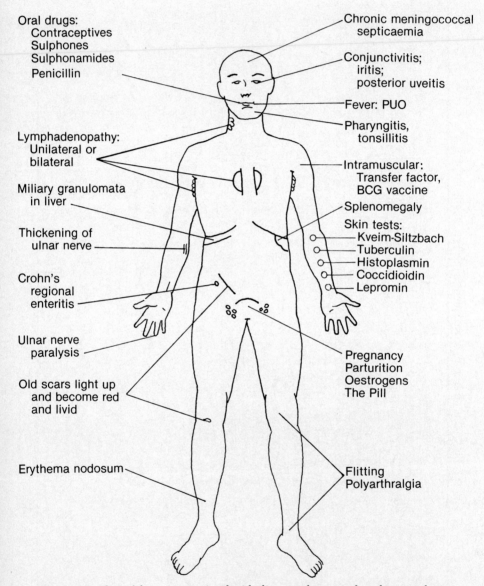

Oral drugs:
  Contraceptives
  Sulphones
  Sulphonamides
  Penicillin

Chronic meningococcal
  septicaemia

Conjunctivitis;
  iritis;
  posterior uveitis

Fever: PUO

Pharyngitis,
  tonsillitis

Lymphadenopathy:
  Unilateral or
  bilateral

Intramuscular:
  Transfer factor,
  BCG vaccine

Miliary granulomata
  in liver

Splenomegaly

Skin tests:
  Kveim-Siltzbach
  Tuberculin
  Histoplasmin
  Coccidioidin
  Lepromin

Thickening of
  ulnar nerve

Crohn's
  regional
  enteritis

Ulnar nerve
  paralysis

Old scars light up
  and become red
  and livid

Pregnancy
Parturition
Oestrogens
The Pill

Erythema nodosum

Flitting
Polyarthralgia

Figure 7–3. Clinical features associated with the several causes of erythema nodosum.

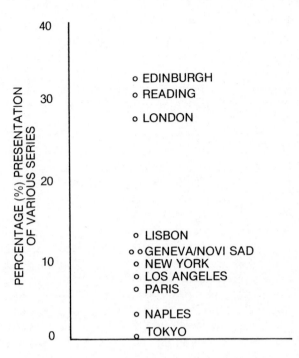

40

PERCENTAGE (%) PRESENTATION OF VARIOUS SERIES

30
○ EDINBURGH
○ READING
○ LONDON

20

Figure 7–4. The worldwide distribution of erythema nodosum due to sarcoidosis is patchy.

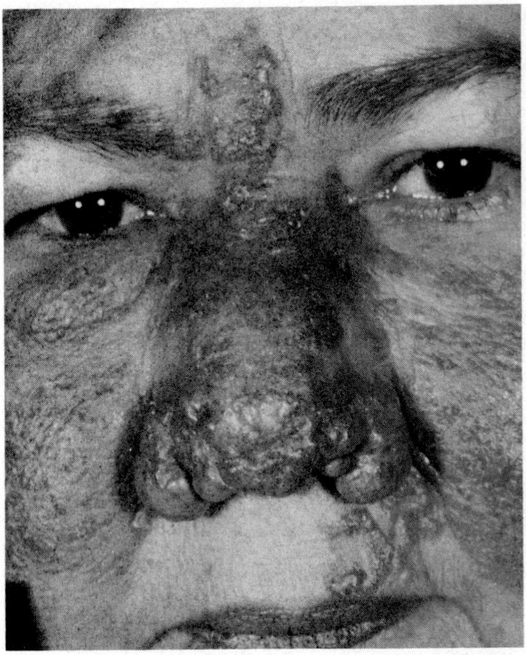

10
○ LISBON
○ ○ GENEVA/NOVI SAD
○ NEW YORK
○ LOS ANGELES
○ PARIS

○ NAPLES
0
○ TOKYO

Figure 7–5. Lupus pernio.

button-like lesions or nodules under the top of the nose to exuberant plaques covering the nose and spreading across both cheeks. There may also be similar plaques or nodules on the scalp (Fig. 7–6; see also color plate 5), eyelids, and pinnae of the ears (Figs. 7–7 and 7–8). Associated sarcoid skin plaques are often seen on the arms, buttocks, and thighs (Fig. 7–9). In our series of 818 patients, 147 had various skin lesions including 35 with lupus pernio.[7]

Whereas sarcoidosis overall usually presents in three-fourths of those under 40 years old, lupus pernio usually presents in three-fourths of those over 40 (Table 7–4). It is twice as common in females as in males and is predominately found in those from the West Indies. It is associated with chronic fibrotic sarcoidosis in many other systems. Compared with sarcoidosis overall, lupus pernio has a closer affinity with sarcoidosis of the upper respiratory tract (SURT), bone cysts, lacrimal gland involvement, and renal sarcoidosis. It was less often associated with erythema nodosum than in the overall series (Table 7–5).

Lupus pernio is an indicator of chronic fibrotic sarcoidosis. It develops insidiously and progresses indolently over the years. It is complicated by nasal ulceration and septal perforation, which may be disastrously aggravated by the well-meaning intervention of nasal and plastic surgeons. Intrathoracic pulmonary infiltration progresses to fibrosis with little tendency toward resolution. It is best kept under control by repeated courses of prednisolone and weekly methotrexate.

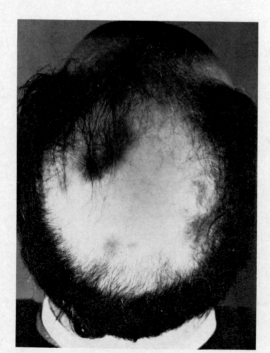

Figure 7–6. Lupus pernio may also involve the scalp.

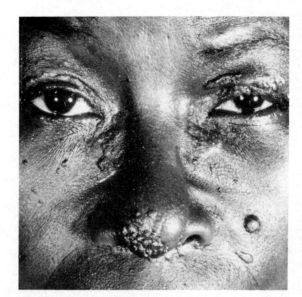

Figure 7–7. Plaques on eyelids and nose.

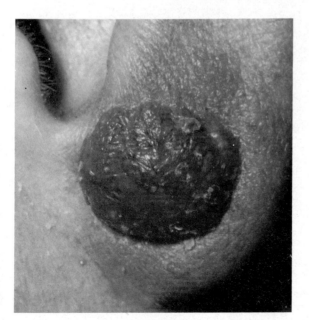

Figure 7–8. Plaque on ear. Keloid following ear piercing.

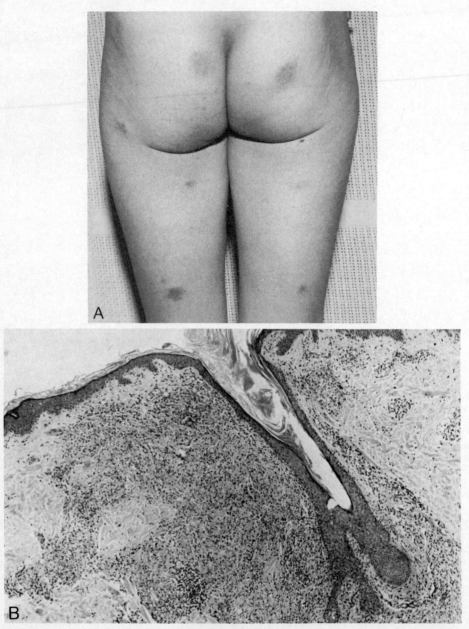

Figure 7–9. *A,* Plaques on trunk. *B,* Plaque of sarcoid tissue. Granulomas extending through the dermis with overlying atrophic epidermis. H & E × 32.

Table 7–4. Age, Sex, and Race of 35 Patients with Lupus Pernio

Feature	Number	%
Age (years)		
21–30	3	9
31–40	10	30
40 +	22	61
Sex		
Female	24	69
Race		
Caucasian	18	51
West Indian	15	43
Other	2	6
Total	35	100

Table 7–5. Features of 818 Patients with Histologically Confirmed Sarcoidosis Compared with 35 Patients with Lupus Pernio Attending the Royal Northern Hospital, London

Feature	Sarcoidosis Overall No. Patients	%	Lupus Pernio No. Patients	%
Women	500	61	24	69
Presentation under 40 years of age	604	74	13	40
Intrathoracic	700	86	29	83
Peripheral lymphadenopathy	225	27	2	6
Splenomegaly	101	12	3	9
Erythema nodosum	251	31	3	9
Other skin lesions	147	21	9	26
Ocular lesions	224	27	8	23
Nervous system	77	9	2	6
SURT	53	6	20	57
Parotid	52	6	4	11
Lacrimal	22	3	3	9
Bone	31	3	6	17
Heart	27	3	0	—
Kidney	10	1	2	6
Positive Kveim-Siltzbach skin test	430/658	65	16/35	46
Negative tuberculin skin test	488/702	70	32/35	91
Hyperglobulinaemia	161/526	31	1	3
Hypercalcaemia	99/547	18	1	3
Corticosteroid therapy	344	42	29	80
Mortality due to				
Sarcoidosis	25	3	0	—
Other causes	23	3	0	—
Total	818	100	35	100

Experimental Model

Lupus pernio is a good experimental therapeutic model because in a single patient there are three features that may be observed and the response to treatment noted serially. The first feature is the very obvious clinical skin lesions. Serial photography records the response to treatment. Effective treatment is followed by improvement in 8 to 12 weeks. The second feature is serial histology of nasal mucosa. Effective treatment will convert sarcoid granulomas into a non-specific inflammatory reaction in the course of six months. Nasal bone erosion, the third feature, is slow to develop and slow to heal, but this may be expected in the course of years.[7]

Therapeutic Response

Corticosteroid therapy and methotrexate are effective treatments of lupus pernio, but, unfortunately, relapses follow withdrawal of treatment. Long-term chloroquine is followed by a moderate response in the course of 9 to 12 months. Anti-tuberculous drugs and levamisole fail to influence lupus pernio (Table 7–6).

Before embarking on a large-scale, long-term, double-blind clinical trial of any new drug for the treatment of sarcoidosis, consider lupus pernio as a therapeutic screen. It will provide helpful data on the clinical response within a few months. To these measures may be added serial measurement of SACE. If there is no clinical or histological response and SACE does not fall as a response to treatment, then it can be assumed that the drug is of little value in overcoming sarcoidosis. It will certainly provide guidance for any prospective expensive long-term trials.

Maculo-papular Eruptions

Transient maculo-papular or vesicular eruptions may herald the onset of the disease, coinciding with acute (rather than chronic) uveitis or parotid gland enlargement. These features are sufficiently alarming and sudden in onset for patients to seek early medical advice and investigation. Intrathoracic

Table 7–6. The Response of Lupus Pernio to Various Drugs

Drug	Dose	Length of Therapy (mon)	Result
Prednisolone	Smallest possible	Shortest possible	Good
Chloroquine	250 mg on alternate days	9	Moderate
Methotrexate	5 mg weekly	3	Very effective
Potassium para-aminobenzoate	12 g daily	12	Slight
Levamisole	150 mg daily	1	Unchanged
Anti-tuberculous	Full	6	Unchanged

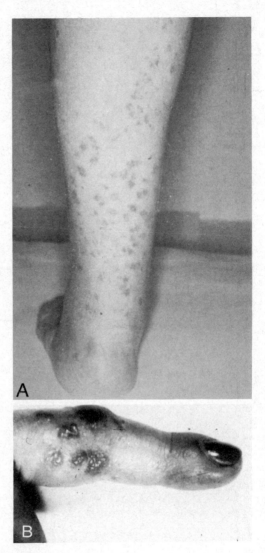

Figure 7–10. A, Transient maculo-papular eruption. B, Transient vesicular eruption.

involvement likewise presents at an earlier stage than in patients with lupus pernio or persistent plaques. The eruption occurs at various sites including the trunk, face, arms, thighs, calves, ears, and fingers (Fig. 7–10). It usually resolves within a month but it may recur with exacerbations of iridocyclitis. It is possible that these transient recurrent multisystem features reflect a circulating immune complex.

Scars

Scars may draw attention to or provide histological evidence of the disease.[8] They include scars of the abdomen or neck, cutaneous venesection

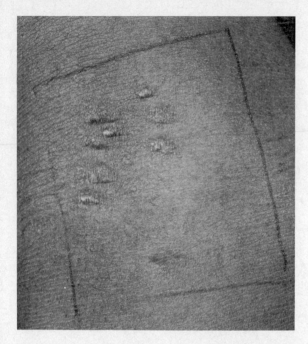

Figure 7–11. Scar at vene-section site.

Figure 7–12. Sarcoid keloid.

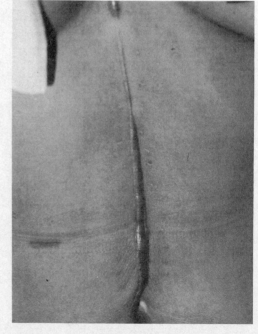

(Figs. 7–11 and 7–12), and tuberculin skin test sites. In all instances these previously atrophic scars suddenly become purple and livid, proclaiming some inflammatory change, and biopsy reveals active sarcoid tissue. There is no explanation for this phenomenon, first noted by Löfgren,[5] in which the sarcoid process seems to creep into and light up these scars, but it suggests a hypersensitivity reaction akin to erythema nodosum and may indicate a circulating immune complex. Inoculation sites such as Mantoux test sites may also contain sarcoid tissue, so they should be scrutinised in the same way as Kveim sites after a month for evidence of palpable nodules. Intrathoracic involvement appears to be longstanding, suggesting that the reaction in the scars is not an initial manifestation of the disease but rather an exacerbation late in its course. Some patients have learned to anticipate an exacerbation of iritis when their scars become livid and inflamed. The scar phenomenon is also observed at the onset of erythema nodosum, but it is then a transient and early feature rather than longstanding and recurrent.[3]

Plaques

Plaques are of various size and distribution and range in colour from red to brown. They may be subcutaneous with an overlying thin epidermis. Lesions may be psoriasiform, telangiectatic, or associated with alopecia (see Figs. 7–7 through 7–9).

REFERENCES

1. James DG. Sarcoidosis of the skin. *In* Fitzpatrick TB (ed.): Dermatology in General Medicine, 3rd ed. New York, McGraw Hill. 1984.
2. James DG, Thomson AD, Willcox A. Erythema nodosum as a manifestation of sarcoidosis. Lancet ii:218, 1956.
3. James DG, Studdy PR. Colour Atlas of Respiratory Disorders. London, Wolfe Medical Publications. 1982.
4. James DG, Neville E, Siltzbach LE, et al. A worldwide review of sarcoidosis. Ann NY Acad Sci. 278:321, 1976.
5. Löfgren S. Primary pulmonary sarcoidosis. Acta Med Scand. 145:424, 1953.
6. Besnier E. Lupus pernio de la face. Ann Derm Syph (Paris). 10:333, 1889.
7. James DG. Lupus pernio. *In* Chretien J, Marsac J, Saltiel JC (eds): Proc 9th Internat Conf Sarcoidosis. Paris, Pergamon Press. p 465, 1983.
8. James DG, Thomson AD. Dermatological aspects of sarcoidosis. Quart J Med. 28:109, 1959.

8

Sarcoidosis of the Heart

The lungs, eyes, skin, and reticulo-endothelial system are major sites of involvement of sarcoidosis, whereas the heart, central nervous system, bone, kidney, and salivary glands are clinically seen to be involved in less than 10 per cent of patients. Myocardial sarcoidosis produces significant symptoms in less than 5 per cent of patients, although cardiac lesions are noted in as many as 20 per cent of autopsy cases. The discrepancy between the incidence of clinical and autopsy involvement of the heart arises because of the difficulty in detecting it clinically. It is suspected when a patient with pulmonary ocular or cutaneous sarcoidosis develops arrhythmias or bundle branch block. It should also be considered when the patient develops atrioventricular block, angina, pericarditis, congestive cardiac failure, or cardiomyopathy. Sudden death without previous evidence of a heart lesion may occur.

Cardiac sarcoidosis was confidently diagnosed in only 27 (3 per cent) patients in our clinical series, comprising 18 (2 per cent) with cor pulmonale and 9 (1 per cent) with myocardial disease; the latter group had arrhythmias but one patient developed acute mitral regurgitation and ventricular tachyarrhythmias. Cardiac sarcoidosis remains a submerged part of an iceberg, and we need to dig deeper to uncover latent forms of the disease.

CLINICAL PRESENTATIONS

Fleming and Bailey have analysed a series of 250 patients from the United Kingdom with sarcoid heart disease (229 white, 21 black), 37 of whom died suddenly and the diagnosis was first made at necropsy.[1] Modes of cardiac presentation, often multiple, included arrhythmias (in 71 patients), heart block (in 49), myocardial disease (in 33), simulated myocardial infarction (in 13), and pericarditis (in 6). Features suggesting mitral valve involvement were noted in 48 and aortic valve involvement in 6 patients. There was a mortality of 43 per cent despite steroids in 24 patients and pacemakers in 5. The main causes of death were cardiomyopathy, heart block, and arrhythmias.

Sarcoid heart disease occurs with equal sex frequency in the 40-year age group in the United Kingdom and in the U.S.[2] but appears to be commoner

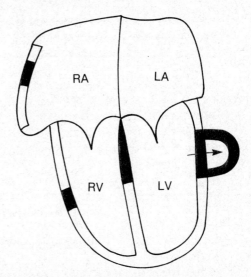

Figure 8–1. Sites of cardiac granulomas due to sarcoidosis.

in older women in Japan.[3] Sites of involvement are most frequently the bundle of His, left ventricle, right ventricle, and, infrequently, the right atrium (Fig. 8–1). Left ventricular involvement leads to congestive cardiac failure, dysrhythmias, and aneurysm formation.

PULMONARY HYPERTENSION

Pulmonary hypertension is a well-recognised complication of pulmonary sarcoidosis. It was noted in 27 (3 per cent) patients in the Royal Northern Hospital series. It may be due to longstanding pulmonary fibrosis or to pulmonary vasculitis; if due to the latter then steroid therapy may reverse the pulmonary hypertension with a fall to normal pulmonary pressure.[4] Rizzato and colleagues have correlated pulmonary hypertension by right heart haemodynamics using Swan-Ganz flow-directed catheters with non-invasive M-mode echocardiography.[5] Haemodynamic studies showed resting pulmonary hypertension in most patients with hilar adenopathy with or without pulmonary infiltration (Stages 1 and 2). Increased right ventricular anterior wall thickness by echocardiography was a helpful non-invasive method of detecting pulmonary hypertension even when the electrocardiogram was normal. In this study echocardiography revealed normal valves for the left atrium and left ventricle.

SUDDEN DEATH

Sudden death in apparently healthy young adults is regrettably too frequent. The Royal Air Force faced this with deep concern and responsibility and arranged a most searching investigation of its aircrew with a past history of sarcoidosis. It is fortunate to relate that cardiac sarcoidosis was not uncovered by these extensive tests of cardiac function.

Fleming and Bailey noted sudden death in 37 (15 per cent) patients in their series.[1] Necropsy studies in the U.S.[2] and Japan[3] (Table 8–1) reveal major similarities in two distinctive ethnic groups. Cardiac sarcoidosis frequently presented with heart block or Stokes-Adams syncope, most commonly in those aged 40 years and older. The prognosis was gloomy, with a duration of less than four years between the recognised onset and death (Figs. 8–2 and 8–3).

DIAGNOSTIC TESTS

Electrocardiography (ECG)

Conventional ECGs only provide crude diagnostic help, perhaps sufficient to arouse suspicion and lead to further investigation and treatment. Routine ECGs selectively used in sarcoidosis clinics at the Mount Sinai Hospital, New York City,[6] and at London's Central Middlesex Hospital[7] disclosed asymptomatic ECG abnormalities in about 10 to 15 per cent of patients with sarcoidosis. However, studies in Helsinki comparing other monitors of disease activity indicate that it is virtually impossible to decide whether these abnormalities are due to sarcoidosis or other diseases.

Electrocardiography with exercise or with 24-hour ambulatory tapes may uncover transient dysrhythmias. Intracardial ECGs and His bundle electrograms may occasionally provide further evidence of myocardial sarcoidosis.

Table 8–1. Features of Cardiac Sarcoidosis in Britain, Japan, and the US

	United Kingdom*	US†	Japan‡
Necropsies	65	113	42
% women	50	50	33
Age	43	40	Over 40
% diagnosed in life	83	27–62	12
Onset to death (years)	1–20	2–4	2
Stokes-Adams attacks	—	22%	18%
Heart block	Majority	27%	Majority

*Data from Fleming HA, Bailey SM. Sarcoid heart disease. J Roy Coll Phys (London). 15:245, 1981.

†Data from Roberts WC, McAllister HA, Ferrous VJ: Sarcoidosis of the heart. Am J Med. 62:86, 1977.

‡Data from Matsui Y, Iwai K, Iachibana T, Furuie T, Shigematou N, Izumi T, Homma AH, Mikomi R, Hongo O, Hiraga Y, Yamamoto M. Clinico-pathological study of fatal myocardial sarcoidosis. Ann N Y Acad Sci. 278:455, 1976.

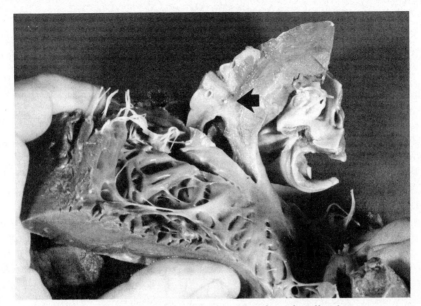

Figure 8–2. Heart showing fibrosis (arrow) involving bundle of His. × 2.

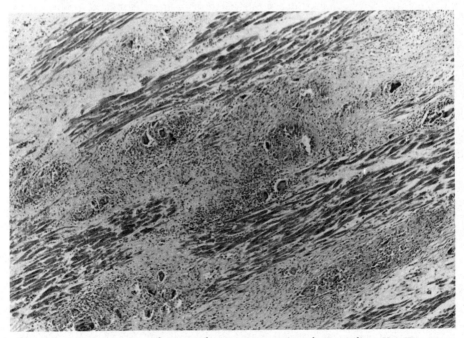

Figure 8–3. Numerous granulomas with extensive scarring of myocardium H & E × 50.

Echocardiography

This non-invasive technique may disclose right ventricular anterior wall thickness, which is good evidence of pulmonary hypertension.[5]

Thallium-201 Imaging

Myocardial uptake of a potassium analogue, thallium-201, from the extracellular space represents the net result of continuous extraction and release of thallium-201 by myocardial cells. After injection, normal myocardial cells accumulate thallium-201. Peak concentration is reached more slowly in poorly perfused zones than in normal zones, and clearance is more rapid from normal zones. The pulmonary uptake of thallium-201 has been related to an increase in pulmonary capillary wedge pressure during exercise and a subsequent increase in pulmonary blood flow.[8]

Sharma advocates resting thallium-201 myocardial scans, which show focal defects in one-third of patients with sarcoidosis.[9] In a series of 35 patients with multisystem disease, 12 (34 per cent) were abnormal, 5 had focal left ventricular defects, 10 had abnormal right ventricular uptake, and 3 patients showed both defects. On stress imaging, all left ventricular defects decreased in size; this effect is unique and the opposite of that noted with coronary artery disease. Right ventricular uptake appears to correlate with the severity of pulmonary involvement. Two patients with left ventricular defects were followed serially to judge the response to steroids; the myocardial defect diminished in one patient but was unchanged in the other.

Fox and Israel[10] have investigated angina in sarcoidosis and characterised a group in which abnormal thallium scans are associated with normal coronary arteriograms.

Cardiac Biopsy

Cardiac biopsy is easily performed by those accustomed to cardiac catheterisation, and it can be done at the same time as catheterisation of the left or right side of the heart. It is recommended by Japanese workers as an aid to the diagnosis of myocardial sarcoidosis when serial changes show worsening of the electrocardiogram or vector cardiography reveals disturbances of conduction.[11] However, they did not find it helpful in assessing treatment.

PROGNOSIS AND TREATMENT

Vigorous steroid therapy and anti-arrhythmic drugs are the sheet anchor of treatment, but the results are not very impressive. A recent Japanese study provides a long-term follow-up of 33 patients in whom permanent pacemakers had been implanted for A-V block.[12] There were 19 cardiac deaths with a survival period of 25 ± 23 months. Out of 12 sudden deaths, 9 patients had not received steroid therapy. Seven deaths were due to congestive cardiac failure.

REFERENCES

1. Fleming HA, Bailey SM. Sarcoid heart disease. J Roy Coll Phys (London). 15:245, 1981.
2. Roberts WC, McAllister HA, Ferrous VJ. Sarcoidosis of the heart. Am J Med. 62:86, 1977.
3. Matsui Y, Iwai K, Tachibana T, Furuie T, Shigematou N, Izumi T, Homma AH, Mikami R, Hongo O, Hiraga Y, Yamamoto M. Clinico-pathological study of fatal myocardial sarcoidosis. Ann N Y Acad Sci. 278:455, 1976.
4. Davies J, Nellen M, Goodwin JF. Reversible pulmonary hypertension in sarcoidosis. Postgrad Med J. 58:282, 1982.
5. Rizzato G, Pezzano A, Bertoli L, Merlini R, Sala G, Montanari G, Lo Cicero S, Conti F. Involvement of the heart in sarcoidosis: echocardiographic and haemodynamic study. In Chretien J, Marsac J, Saltiel JC (eds): Proc 9th Internat Conf Sarcoidosis. Paris, Pergamon Press. p 618, 1983.
6. Stein E, Stimmel B, Siltzbach LE. Clinical course of cardiac sarcoidosis. Ann N Y Acad Sci. 278:470, 1976.
7. Mikhail JR, Mitchell DN, Sutherland I, McNicol MW. Sarcoidosis presenting in a district general hospital. In Jones Williams W, Davies BH (eds): Proc 8th Internat Conf Sarcoidosis. Cardiff, Alpha and Omega Press. p 532, 1980.
8. Berger HJ, Zaret BL. Nuclear cardiology. N Engl J Med. 305:799, 1981.
9. Sharma OP. Thallium-201 imaging in the management of myocardial sarcoidosis. In Chretien J, Marsac J, Saltiel JC (eds): Proc 9th Internat Conf Sarcoidosis. Paris, Pergamon Press. p 619, 1983.
10. Fox HB, Israel HL. Myocardial sarcoidosis: a cause of praecordial pain. Bull Europ Physiopath Resp. 17:82, 1981.
11. Numao Y, Sekiguchi M, Furuie T, Matsui Y, Izumi T, Mikami R. A study of cardiac involvement in 963 cases of sarcoidosis by ECG and endomyocardial biopsy. In Jones Williams W, Davies BH (eds): Sarcoidosis. Cardiff, Alpha and Omega Press. p 697, 1980.
12. Sekiguchi M, Suda T, Furuie T, Matsui Y, Numao Y, Osada H, Tachibana T, Yamamoto M, Mikami R. Long-term prognosis of cardiac sarcoidosis patients with permanent pacemaker implantation. In Chretien J, Marsac J, Saltiel JC (eds): Proc 9th Internat Conf Sarcoidosis. Paris, Pergamon Press. p 658, 1983.

9

Lymphoreticular System

LYMPH NODES AND SPLEEN

There are so many different causes of granulomas in lymph nodes that involvement by sarcoidosis demands a synthesis of a compatible multisystem clinical picture, chest radiographical changes, and histological features. This appears to be rigid and demanding, but unless these standards are maintained there will be confusion with numerous infections, neoplasms, reticuloses, mineral particles, Crohn's disease, primary biliary cirrhosis, Whipple's disease, dermatopathic and silicone lymphadenopathy, and drug-induced and allergic granulomatous lymphadenopathies (Table 9–1).

Lymph involvement in sarcoidosis most commonly affects the pulmonary hilar glands and is practically always bilateral (BHL) (see Chapter 5). In this chapter we are concerned with peripheral lymphadenopathy and involvement of the spleen.

Peripheral lymphadenopathy was noted in 225 of 818 patients (27 per cent) and splenomegaly in 101 patients (12 per cent) in our own series as compared to the worldwide series of 3,676 patients, in which peripheral lymphadenopathy and splenomegaly were present in 1,031 patients (28 per cent) (see Table 4–1).

Involvement of scalene lymph nodes is common and has been used for blind biopsy confirmation of the diagnosis (see Chapter 3). Other commonly affected sites include the axillae and the inguinal, iliac, lumbar, and epitrochlear groups. The affected glands are usually discrete, painless, and only moderately enlarged. Gross enlargement is unusual. Clinically, Hodgkin's disease must be excluded, but as widespread lymph gland enlargement is unusual, distinction from other reticuloses is rarely a problem. As always, tuberculosis must also be considered.

Splenomegaly is usually slight and silent, although rarely it may be gross and may necessitate removal for pressure symptoms and even spontaneous rupture. Asymptomatic involvement of a normal-sized spleen is common. It was present in 17 of 36 (47 per cent) patients who underwent splenic puncture for diagnosis, thus emphasizing the widespread multisystem nature of sarcoidosis. Splenomegaly may be associated with signs of hypersplenism, pancytopaenia, thrombocytopaenia, purpura, and haemolytic anaemia.

118

Table 9–1. Disorders Associated With Granulomatous Lymph Nodes

Infections		Other
Mycobacteria M. tuberculosis M. kansasii M. xenopei M. avium M. intracellulare M. scrofulaceum M. leprae *Bacteria* Brucella sp. Francisella tularensis Pseudomonas mallei Propioni sp. Yersinia sp.	*Spirochaetes* Treponema pallidum *Fungi* Blastomyces sp. Coccidioides immitis Histoplasma capsulatum Cryptococcus neoformans *Protozoa* Leishmania sp. Toxoplasma sp. *Other* Cat scratch disease Schistosoma sp. Filaria sp.	*Chemicals* Beryllium *Immunologic upset* Sarcoidosis Crohn's disease Primary biliary cirrhosis Hypogammaglobulinaemia Whipple's disease Immune complexes *Enzyme defect* Chronic granulomatous disease of childhood *Neoplasia* Reticulosis Carcinoma

A notable feature of sarcoidosis in lymphoid and other tissues is the combination of old scarring and the persistence of discrete "fresh" cellular granulomas. The granulomas are widely distributed throughout the node and primarily start in the interfollicular T cell zones (Fig. 9–1). Coalescence and fusion of the granulomas are uncommon. Cell inclusions are common and are suggestive, but not diagnostic, of sarcoidosis (see Chapter 3).

Let us now consider the differential diagnosis, in particular as it affects the histopathologist (Table 9–2).

INFECTIONS

Mycobacterium tuberculosis

The granulomas frequently involve only part of the lymph node, usually coalesce, and frequently surround a large central area of caseation.

In patients with a high degree of immunity against tuberculosis, the granulomas remain discrete and non-caseating and may be indistinguishable from sarcoidosis (Fig. 9–2). The mycobacteria must then be detected by special staining and by culture. All tissue-labelled sarcoidosis must be cultured for mycobacteria and care taken to adjust culture temperatures to meet the requirements of various species.

Enlargement of lymph nodes is a feature of primary tuberculosis infecting hilar lymph nodes or *Mycobacterium bovis* infecting cervical and mesenteric lymph nodes (see Table 15–3). Secondary or re-infected tuberculosis does not cause enlargement of lymph nodes. The spleen is involved when there is miliary spread from both primary and secondary infection.

Mycobacterium balnei, which causes swimming pool granulomas, infects axillary and inguinal lymph nodes. The draining lymph nodes are heavily involved with extensive caseation, whereas the primary skin infection may

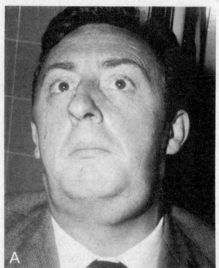

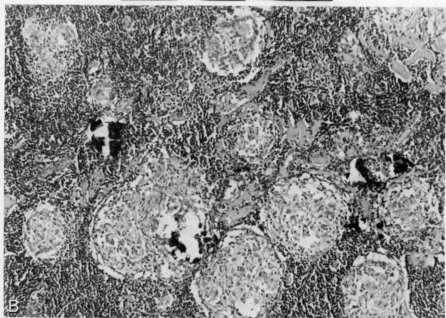

Figure 9–1. *A*, Sarcoid lymphadenopathy. *B*, Sarcoid granulomas in lymph node. Note Schaumann's bodies. H & E × 120.

Table 9–2. Cellular and Other Features of Lymph Node Granulomas

Disease	Focal Granulomas	Necrosis	Polymorphs	Plasma Cells	Eosinophils	Schaumann's Bodies	Other Features
Sarcoidosis	+++	– to ±	–	–	–	80%	Calcification rare
Tuberculosis	+++ (confluent)	+ to +++ Caseation	–	–	–	<2%	Calcification frequent
Tuberculoid leprosy	±	–	–	–	–	–	–
Hodgkin's disease	+ to +++	–	+	+	++	–	Tumour cells
Chronic beryllium disease	+++	– to ++	–	–	–	60%	–
Histoplasmosis }	++	+ to +++	+ to +++	+	+	–	Calcification frequent
Cryptococcosis }							
Toxoplasmosis }	+ to ++	±	±	+	+	–	Small isolated foci of histiocytes
Leishmaniasis }	+	–	–	++	–	–	–
Infectious mononucleosis (EBV)				++			
Syphilis	±+	– to +++	–	+++	–	–	Vasculitis
Bacterial	+	– to +++	+ to +++	++	±+	–	Yersinia or Propioni abscess

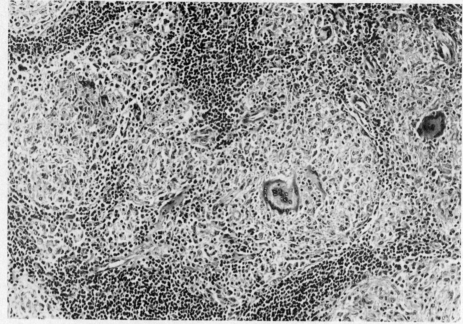

Figure 9–2. Coalescing granulomas in tuberculosis lymph node (Ziehl-Neelsen stain and culture positive). H & E × 150. Note that tuberculous granulomas are not always caseous.

be inconspicuous. The microscopic picture is similar to that of *M. kansasii, M. xenopei, M. avium,* and *M. scrofulaceum,* but plasma cells are more evident.

Mycobacterium leprae[2]

Lymphadenopathy is a feature of lepromatous leprosy. There are prominent large multinucleated lepra cells containing easily identified bacilli. Epithelioid cell granulomas are not a feature of lepromatous leprosy but rather of tuberculoid leprosy, in which lymphadenopathy is less of a feature.

Brucella

There are loose collections of macrophages admixed with polymorphs, plasma cells, and occasional eosinophils. The granulomas are not compact, as in sarcoidosis, and Langhans'-type giant cell and caseation are inconspicuous or exceptional.

Yersinia

These organisms cause granulomatous mesenteric lymphadenitis. Numerous epithelioid cells are arranged around many areas of necrosis containing eosinophils and numerous polymorphs to give the picture of a pseudo-abscess. Discrete focal granulomas are unusual. The same features are seen in the lymph nodes in cat scratch disease,[3] which may be causally related (Fig. 9–3).

Francisella tularensis

This is acquired from rabbits, hares, and squirrels, possibly via tick bites. The histology is similar to that of *Yersinia* infection, with palisading epithelioid cells surrounding a pseudo-abscess.

Pseudomonas mallei

This causes glanders in horses but rarely affects humans. The histology is similar to that of *Yersinia* infections, with considerable necrosis surrounded by epithelioid and a few giant cells.

Treponema pallidum

Generalised lymphadenopathy is a feature of secondary syphilis. The distinguishing features are the excess of plasma cells, paucity of giant cells,

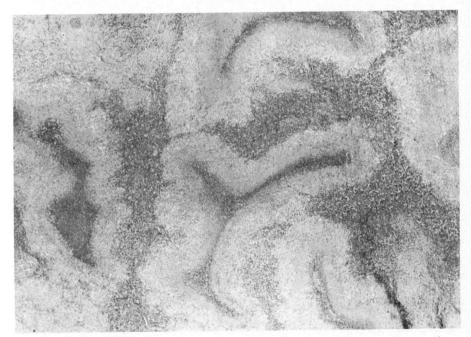

Figure 9–3. Stellate necrosis with surrounding epithelioid cells, characteristic of cat scratch disease. H & E × 20.

and lack of necrosis. (If the lymph node has been subjected to the Jarisch-Herxheimer reaction, then necrosis is evident and the disease may resemble caseating tuberculosis.)

Toxoplasma[4]

This is one cause of glandular fever. The lymph node appearance rarely may be indistinguishable from that of sarcoidosis, but scattered small groups of macrophage giving a starry-sky appearance are more usual (Fig. 9–4).

Leishmania

Generalised lymphadenopathy is associated with hepatosplenomegaly. Single or focal collections of macrophages are seen to contain Leishman-Donovan bodies. Unless special stains are done, there may be superficial confusion with sarcoidosis or tuberculosis.

Schistosoma

Schistosoma ova may be embedded within an epithelioid cell granuloma. Giant cells are of the multinucleate giant cell type, and eosinophils are

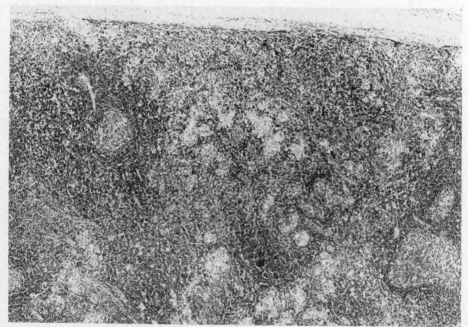

Figure 9–4. Toxoplasmosis showing isolated and small foci of macrophages. H & E × 120.

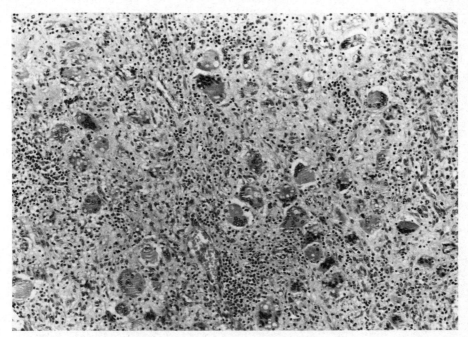

Figure 9–5. Histoplasmosis present in giant cells with diffuse macrophage and lympho-cytic interpretation; compact sarcoid granulomas are rare. H & E × 80.

conspicuous. In a later stage, calcified ova may be buried in fibrous nodules; they are distinguished from Schaumann's bodies because they lack the aggregated spherules and crystalline material.

Histoplasma capsulatum

This causes hilar and peripheral lymphadenopathy. Histoplasmosis mimics sarcoidosis clinically and in the chest radiograph and in lymph node tissue sections. The organism is observed within macrophages and epithe-lioid cells with PAS and silver staining (Fig. 9–5). Similar superficial confusion may be associated with *Coccidioides immitis* and *Cryptococcus neoformans*. Caseous necrosis may occur, so that first glance histology would favor tuberculosis rather than sarcoidosis.

CHRONIC GRANULOMATOUS DISEASE OF CHILDHOOD

This is characterized by a deficiency of oxidative enzymes in both leucocytes and macrophages, resulting in multisystem infections by a variety of organisms, in particular "opportunistic" infections (see Chapter 14).

Tuberculoid granulomas varying from non-caseating sarcoid-like lesions to the common large necrotic abscesses or tuberculous-like foci are frequent. *M. tuberculosis* is absent.

NEOPLASIA

Sarcoid granulomas may occur in lymph nodes draining a variety of tumours (Fig. 9–6). They are identical on light and electron microscopy to those seen in sarcoidosis,[5] e.g., carcinoma of the breast, stomach, thyroid, and ovaries and sometimes within such tumours. In some rare tumours, e.g., pinealoma, dysgerminoma and seminoma, granulomas are a usual feature within the tumours. It is emphasized that these are local reactions probably caused by products of tumour necrosis, although the possibility of an immune response has been considered.[6]

Sarcoid-like granulomas may be admixed with the Hodgkin's tumour tissue and even seen in lymphoid tissue independent of the tumour.[7] We have seen a patient with extensive granulomas in the spleen with no associated tumour whose cervical glands were replaced by Hodgkin's tissue without granulomas. The presence of eosinophils in the granulomas of Hodgkin's disease is a common feature, but they are absent in the granulomas of sarcoidosis.[8] The localised nature of granulomas and the presence of eosinophils are therefore of value in distinguishing the two conditions (Table 9–3).

SARCOIDOSIS AND MALIGNANT TUMOURS

Care must be taken to exclude local epithelioid cell reaction to tumour (see previous discussion) before accepting the co-existence of sarcoidosis and

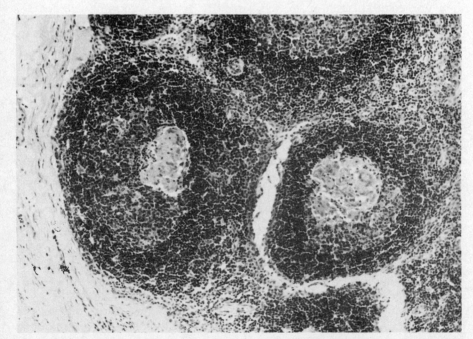

Figure 9–6. Isolated sarcoid granulomas in lymph node–draining carcinoma of the rectum. H & E × 80.

Table 9–3. Comparison Between Sarcoidosis and Hodgkin's Disease

Feature	Sarcoidosis	Hodgkin's Disease
Age (years)	20–40	20–40
Male:female	Equal	3:1
Weight loss	Rare	Common
Splenomegaly	Rare	Frequent
Segmental lymph nodes	Infrequent	Frequent
Erythema nodosum	Frequent	Rare
Gut symptoms	Absent	Common
Pruritus	Absent	Common
Bone lesions	"Punched out" phalangeal cysts	Sclerotic lesions of spine and pelvis
Sclerotic lesions	No	Mixed sclerotic/osteolytic in 16%
Leucocytosis, lymphopenia, and eosinophilia	Not a feature	May be present
Hilar lymphadenopathy	Bilateral	Bilateral or unilateral
Hilar gland pressure symptoms	No	Yes
Pulmonary infiltration	Common	Uncommon
Pulmonary infiltration followed by hilar adenopathy	Never	Yes
Pleural effusion	Rare	Common
Skin lesions	Distinctive histology	Specific histology with eosinophilia
Secondary infections	Rare	Common
Abdominal lymphangiogram	Normal	Abnormal
Delayed-type hypersensitivity	Depressed	Depressed
Immunoglobulins	Abnormal	Normal
Kveim-Siltzbach test	Positive	Negative
Radiotherapy	Unhelpful	Curative
Corticosteroids	Therapy of choice	Helpful
Immunosuppressive regimens	Not indicated	Indicated
Prognosis	Good	Guarded

malignant tumours. Both the Kveim test[9] and SACE[10] estimation are of value in making the distinction.

There have been a number of isolated case reports of an association between sarcoidosis and malignant lymphoma, including Hodgkin's disease[11, 12] lymphosarcoma,[13] mycosis fungoides,[14] and reticulosarcoma.[15] It has been suggested that the altered T cell function in sarcoidosis, like immunosuppressant drug therapy, may be a predisposing factor.[16] In a large series of 2,544 sarcoid patients,[17] the incidence of malignant lymphoma was claimed to be 11 times the expected rate, but the diagnosis in many of these cases is in dispute.[18, 19]

It has also been claimed that the incidence of lung cancer, but not cancer at other sites, is three times the expected incidence, but again these figures are disputed.[18, 19]

We therefore conclude that the association of sarcoidosis and malignancy is fortuitous rather than established.

MINERAL PARTICLES

Silica. Even in the absence of overt exposure and with no evidence of silicosis, a granulomatous reaction to silica is a common finding in mediastinal and other lymph nodes and in inguinal glands following road accidents. The brightly birefringent crystalline particles are readily identified with polarized light (which is essential for all examinations of granuloma-containing material). The highly fibrogenic silica is surrounded by whorled fibrotic nodules.

Talc. This persisting indigestible material stimulates macrophage production, resulting in focal collections of cells, including foreign body giant cells. Talc is recognized by its birefringence and the plate-like shape of the crystals (see Fig. 5–7).

Beryllium. Chronic beryllium disease closely mimics sarcoidosis, but enlargement of hilar lymph nodes is rare. The epithelioid cell granulomas are histologically indistinguishable from those of sarcoidosis and can affect any organ. Diagnosis is determined by a history of exposure, by the finding of beryllium in the tissues, and by a positive *in vitro* lymphocyte transformation test (see Chapter 5).

IMMUNOLOGICAL DISORDERS AND LYMPH NODE GRANULOMAS

Immunoblastic (Angioimmunoblastic) Lymphadenopathy.[20] It is characterized by replacement of the architecture by immunoblasts (primitive plasma, B lymphocyte cells) with proliferation of small blood vessels, frequently showing small epithelioid cell foci. The presence of multinucleated plasma cells, eosinophils, and polymorphs may cause confusion with Hodgkin's disease. The disease is associated with polyclonal hypergammaglobulinaemia. It has a poor prognosis.

Hypogammaglobulinaemia. This rare immune deficiency state may affect both B and T cell areas of lymph nodes with loss of follicles and paracortical cells, respectively. Scanty small foci of epithelioid cells may occasionally be seen but could well be due to infection by unidentified organisms, in particular toxoplasmosis, to which these patients are particularly prone.

ALIMENTARY TRACT LYMPH NODE GRANULOMAS (see Chapter 11)

Crohn's Disease. Lymph nodes may show isolated granulomas in about 20 per cent of cases. Necrosis is uncommon, Schaumann's bodies are rare, and there may be extensive oedema and inflammatory hyperplasia.

Primary Biliary Cirrhosis. Granulomas in portal tract lymph nodes may be seen in primary biliary cirrhosis. They occur as isolated small granulomas, unassociated with necrosis. There may be superficial diagnostic confusion when granulomas are found in abdominal lymph nodes, liver, and lung.

Other Causes of Granulomas in Mesenteric Lymph Nodes. Cholegranulomatous lymphadenitis (CL), cystic pneumatosis (CP), and Whipple's disease (WD) may also cause granulomas in mesenteric lymph nodes. CL is distinguished by the presence of bile and mucoproteins within small diffuse foci of foamy macrophages, which only rarely take the form of sarcoid epithelioid cell granulomas. The changes result from leakage of gallbladder contents in longstanding chronic cholecystitis. Similar changes are occasionally found within the liver in relation to obstructed bile ducts and may then cause confusion with granulomas found in primary biliary cirrhosis. CP is an ill understood phenomenon in which gas cysts (unassociated with gas-producing organisms) affect the intestinal wall and draining lymph nodes. Macrophage and epithelioid cells surround the cysts, sometimes with the formation of Langhans'-type giant cells with occasional eosinophils. Similar changes may occur around lipid-containing cysts in WD, which is characterised by prominent PAS-positive staining histiocytes, as in the interstitial mucosa (see Fig. 11–6).

MISCELLANEOUS GRANULOMATOUS LYMPHADENOPATHY

Dermatopathic lymphadenitis. Lymph nodes draining chronic skin diseases may contain epithelioid and Langhans'-type giant cell granulomas mixed with sinus histiocytes and distinguished by the presence of melanin and lipid pigments and prominent eosinophils (Fig. 9–7). The alternative name *lipo-melanic reticulosis* emphasises these pseudo-lymphomatous features.

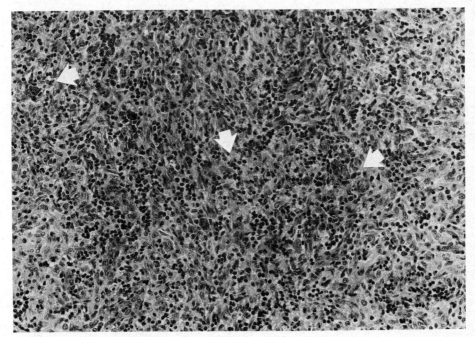

Figure 9–7. Dermatopathic lymphadenopathy, showing diffuse melanin-containing macrophages (arrows) with pseudolymphomatous background. H & E × 120.

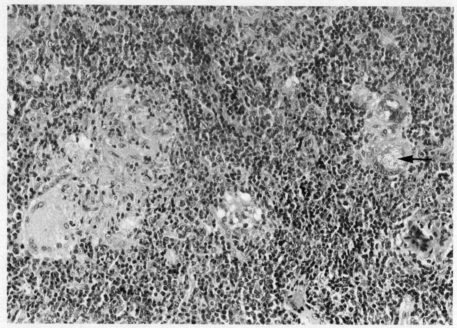

Figure 9–8. Silicon granulomas showing macrophage foci with foreign body–type giant cells containing refractile silicon particles (*arrow*). H & E × 80.

Silicone Lymphadenopathy.[21] This is a reaction to silicone particles in lymph nodes draining prostheses. Focal collections of macrophages and giant cells superficially mimic sarcoid granulomas but are distinguished by the presence of faintly birefringent organic silicon (Fig. 9–8).

Lymphangiographic Lymphadenopathy. Reactive changes to commonly used radio-opaque solutions such as Lipiodol are the source of lipogranulomas. Macrophages, foreign bodies, giant cells, and eosinophils accumulate around lipid-filled cysts. Similar changes may follow the use of oily media for "depot" injections.

Drug-induced Granulomatous Lymph Nodes. Chief among these are anticonvulsant drugs, particularly hydantoin lymphadenopathy, and anti-inflammatory drugs such as phenylbutazone. The changes mimic lymphomas and, in particular, immunoblastic lymphomas; these occasional isolated giant cells and small macrophage foci seldom, if ever, mimic the widespread focal granulomas of sarcoidosis.

REFERENCES

1. Selroos O. Fine needle aspiration biopsy of the spleen in diagnosis of sarcoidosis. Ann NY Acad Sci. 278:517, 1976.
2. Ridley MJ, Field A. The granuloma in leprosy. An immunoperoxidase study. *In* Chretien J, Marsac J, Saltiel JC (eds): Proc 9th Internat Conf Sarcoidosis. Paris, Pergamon Press. p 567, 1983.

3. Naji AF, Carbonell F, Barker HJ. Cat scratch disease. A report of three new cases, review of the literature and classification of the pathological changes in the lymph nodes during various stages of the disease. Am J Clin Pathol. 38:513, 1962.
4. Dorfman RF, Remington JS. Value of lymph node biopsy in the diagnosis of acute acquired toxoplasmosis. N Engl J Med. 289:878, 1973.
5. Syrjanen KJ. Epithelioid cell granulomas in the lymph nodes draining human cancer. Ultrastructural findings of a breast cancer case. Diag Histopathol. 4:291, 1981.
6. Spector WG, Mariano M. Macrophage behaviour in experimental granulomas. *In* van Furth R (ed): Mononuclear Phagocytes in Immunity, Infection and Pathology. Oxford, Blackwell. p 927, 1975.
7. Lennert K, Mestdach J. Lymphogranulomatosen mit konstant hohem Epithelioidzell gehalt. Virch Archiv Abt A Pathol Anat. 344:1, 1968.
8. Jones Williams W, Jones DL, Whittaker JL. Isolated sarcoid like granulomas in Hodgkin's disease. *In* Jones Williams W, Davies BH (eds): Sarcoidosis. Cardiff, Alpha and Omega Press. p 758, 1980.
9. Atwood WG, Miller RC, Nelson CT. Sarcoidosis and the malignant lymphoreticular diseases. Arch Dermatol. 94:144, 1966.
10. Romer FK, Emmertsen K. Serum angiotensin converting enzyme in malignant lymphomas, leukaemia and multiple myeloma. Br J Cancer 42:314. 1980.
11. Goldfarb BL, Cohen SC. Coexistent disseminated sarcoidosis and Hodgkin's disease. J Am Med Assoc. 211:1625, 1970.
12. Brinker H. Sarcoid reaction and sarcoidosis in Hodgkin's disease and other malignant lymphomata. Br J Cancer. 26:120, 1972.
13. Silver HM, Nachnani G, Breslow A. Lymphosarcoma and sarcoidosis. Am Rev Resp Dis. 96:290, 1967.
14. McFarland JP, Kauh YC, Luscombe HA. Sarcoidosis associated with mycosis fungoides. Arch Dermatol. 114:912, 1978.
15. Buckle RM. Reticulosarcoma complicating sarcoidosis. Tubercle (Lon). 41:213, 1960.
16. Israel HL. Sarcoidosis, malignancy and immunosuppressive therapy. Arch Intern Med. 138:907, 1978.
17. Brinker H, Wilbek E. The incidence of malignant tumours in patients with respiratory sarcoidosis. Br J Cancer. 29:247, 1974.
18. Romer FK. Sarcoidosis and cancer—a critical view. *In* Jones Williams W, Davies BH (eds): Sarcoidosis. Cardiff, Alpha and Omega Press. p 567, 1980.
19. Romer FK. Case 7 1982: Sarcoidosis and cancer (letter). N Engl J Med. 306:1490, 1982.
20. Cullen MH, Stansfeld AG, Olver RTD, Lister TA, Malpas JS. Angioimmunoblastic lymphadenopathy. Report of ten cases and review of the literature. Quart J Med. 48:151, 1979.
21. Christie AJ, Weinberger A, Dietrich M. Silicone lymphadenopathy and synovitis, complications of silicone elastomer finger joint prosthesis. J Am Med Assoc. 237:1463, 1977.

10

Locomotor System

MUSCLE

Whereas asymptomatic involvement of muscle is sufficiently common to make muscle biopsy an accepted method of tissue diagnosis (see Chapter 3, p. 33), symptomatic involvement is distinctly rare.[1, 2] There are two main patterns depending on whether sarcoidosis is of acute or insidious onset. Acute sarcoidosis may present as polymyositis with fever, muscle pains, and tenderness of limb muscles. It is benign and self-limiting, subsiding swiftly with systemic steroids. At this acute stage, muscle biopsy is a fruitful source of sarcoid granulomas; serial sections should be cut through the specimen. (Fig. 10–1).

In the chronic persistent type of sarcoidosis, there may be palpable muscle nodules, muscle wasting and weakness, muscle hypertrophy, and contractures. Electromyography shows non-specific changes; steroid therapy provides relief of symptoms.

Acute Polymyositis

Histological evidence of sarcoid granulomas is most often found when acute polymyositis is associated with erythema nodosum, polyarthralgia, and hilar adenopathy. This syndrome may be part of a circulating immune complex that also involves muscle. This form of multisystem muscle sarcoidosis should not be confused with granulomatous polymyositis, which has a similar histological picture but different clinical features.[3] Granulomatous polymyositis is a slowly progressive muscular disorder that most commonly affects post-menopausal women. It is most important to differentiate sarcoidosis of muscle from muscle involvement found in other diseases, such as tuberculosis, toxoplasmosis, carcinoma, myasthenia gravis, immune-complex disease, rheumatoid arthritis, and dermatomyositis.

Acute polymyositis due to sarcoidosis may also be rapidly progressive, converting a healthy young person into a bedridden incapacitant.[4] This "galloping" form of the disease is very rare, and we have only observed it in black patients from the Caribbean; the focal granulomas are unlikely to be the cause of the extensive myopathy. Considerably more data are needed on the histology, electron microscopy, and biochemistry of the muscles.

132

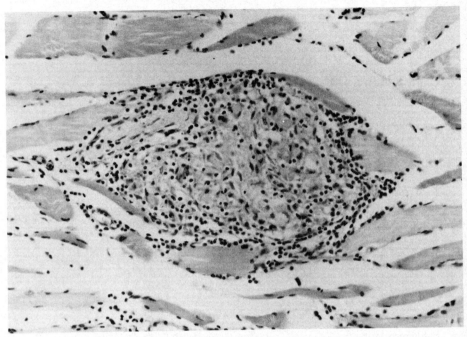

Figure 10–1. Sarcoid granuloma in muscle. H & E × 120.

Chronic Myopathy

Sarcoidosis may be associated with a clinical picture of bilateral weakness and wasting of proximal limb muscles with occasional pseudo-hypertrophy resembling muscular dystrophy.[5] Another report describes three patients, two at autopsy.[6] One showed widespread granulomas in muscles with minor involvement of lungs and hilar lymph nodes. The other showed very few granulomas in only a few muscles associated with a non-specific patchy inflammatory infiltrate, and the lungs showed granulomas and Schaumann's bodies. As in insidious-onset sarcoidosis in other systems, the response to steroid therapy is poor.

Muscle Nodules

Patients with sarcoidosis very rarely also complain of tender muscle nodules.[7] These may vary in size from a pea to a walnut. They are particularly evident in the deltoid muscles. In one of our patients there was complicating rupture of the head of the biceps. In another patient, muscle nodules were a presenting feature. A 5 cm solitary nodule appeared in the left gastrocne- mius muscle, followed 3 years later by a similar nodule at the same site in

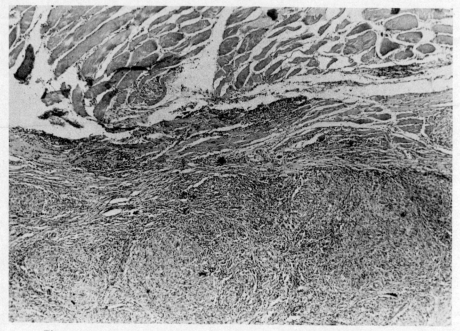

Figure 10–2. Granulomatous muscle nodules, 4 cm in diameter. H & E × 20.

the right leg together with evidence of intrathoracic disease and a positive Kveim test. Both nodules consisted of a mass of sarcoid granulomas (Fig. 10–2).

BONE

Bone involvement by sarcoidosis was recognised soon after the introduction of x-rays,[8–10] its frequency varying in different series (Table 10–1). Even before the introduction of x-rays, Besnier had noted the association of swelling of the fingers with lupus pernio.[11] This association of bone cysts with lupus pernio and other chronic skin lesions continues to be well-recognised. Indeed, bone involvement is rarely found in the absence of skin lesions.[12] The frequency of bone involvement in sarcoidosis varies between 1 and 13 per cent (see Table 10–1). Radiology is a coarse reflection of bone involvement, and only gross changes are apparent. There is evidence of decreased mineral accretion in early sarcoidosis without radiographical changes.[13] Bone sarcoidosis is infrequently reported in sites other than the hands and feet. This is not an observational artifact, since skeletal surveys have been fruitless.[14] In 1972, Bouvier and colleagues reported one case of skull vault sarcoidosis and reviewed six other cases from the world literature,[15] all lytic lesions similar to those in our own patients. Osteoporosis of the nasal bones in association with nasal mucosal sarcoidosis and lupus

Table 10–1. Frequency of Bone Lesions in Large Series of Patients with Sarcoidosis from 10 Cities*

City	Number of Patients With Sarcoidosis	Number of Patients With Bone X-Rays	Bone Lesions No.	Bone Lesions %
London	537	475	19	4
New York	311	139	13	9
Paris	329	165	6	4.5
Los Angeles	150	60	3	4
Tokyo	282	282	5	2
Reading	425	425	5	1
Lisbon	89	89	12	13
Edinburgh	502	502	6	1.2
Novi Sad	285	225	25	11
Geneva	121	121	4	3
Total	3,031	2,483	98	3

*Data from James DG, Neville E, Siltzbach LE, et al. A worldwide review of sarcoidosis. Ann NY Acad Sci. 278:321, 1976.

pernio is well-recognised.[10, 16] Osteolytic lesions may also occur in the long bones[17, 18] and the vertebrae.[19] Sarcoidosis has also been reported in the ribs.[20] Radiodense bone lesions are exceptional.

PERSONAL SERIES

In our series of 29 patients with bone cysts followed for up to 43 years, 19 (66 per cent) were female and 18 (62 per cent) presented in the fourth and fifth decades (Table 10–2). Bone cysts were present in the hands and/or feet in 26 patients, in the nasal bone in 3, and in the hard palate and temporal bone in 1 each.

Table 10–2. Presenting Age, Sex, Race, and Clinical Features of 29 Patients with Osseous Sarcoidosis

Feature	Patients No.	Patients %
Age at Onset (years)		
< 30	6	21
31–40	11	38
41–50	7	24
> 50	5	17
Female	19	66
White	24	83
Black	5	17
Clinical features		
Stiffness	14	48
Pain	13	45
Soft tissue swelling	13	45
Deformity	3	10

Sex, Age, and Race

Nineteen (66 per cent) patients were female, presenting in the fourth and fifth decades in 18 (62 per cent) instances. Twenty-four (83 per cent) patients were white, 20 of whom were English and four Irish, Scottish, Welsh, and Australian, respectively. The remaining five were black West Indians.

Symptoms

About one-half of patients had pain and stiffness of digits, but in only four patients was it sufficient to draw attention to sarcoidosis. Patients with lupus pernio tended to have deformities of the fingers (Fig. 10–3). Soft tissue swelling overlying bone cysts occurred in 13 (45 per cent) patients, preceding radiological diagnosis of bone sarcoidosis for up to four years in 10 patients. In one patient the radiological abnormality was noted six months before the appearance of soft tissue swelling and in another the two events were virtually simultaneous. Thirteen (45 per cent) patients were asymptomatic. One patient with skull vault involvement had painless overlying soft tissue swelling.

Bone Radiology

Lytic lesions occurred in 25 patients. They were either minute cortical defects in phalangeal heads or larger rounded punched-out cysts involving cortex and medulla, most frequently in the heads of middle and proximal phalanges (Fig. 10–4) or less frequently in the metacarpal heads. They were associated with areas of diffuse absorption or destruction of medullary trabeculae (Fig. 10–5). Nasal bone lesions were always small lytic defects on a background of osteoporosis.

Permeative lesions were noted in nine patients. "Tunnelling" of the cortex of the shaft of the phalanx in a proximal direction is followed by remodelling of the cortical and trabecular architecture to give a reticular pattern (Fig. 10–6). The concave shafts become tubular, and cortical structure and shape disappear (Fig. 10–7). In four of the nine patients with permeative lesions there were accompanying lytic lesions. Pressure narrowing of the neck of abnormal phalanges occurred in two patients in association with prolonged soft tissue swelling (Fig. 10–8).

Destructive lesions were observed in three patients. There was rapidly advancing bone involvement with multiple fractures of devitalised cortex and sequestrum formation (Fig. 10–9). There was also secondary joint destruction due to sarcoid lesions in the subchondral bone. In one instance, a periosteal reaction was noted. This is exceptional, for periosteal reaction is

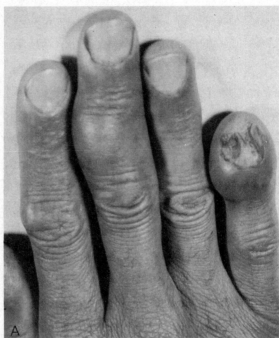

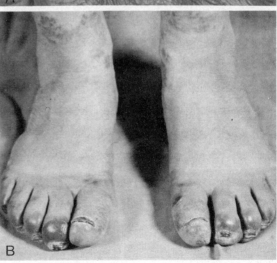

Figure 10–3. Deformities of (A) fingers and (B) toes.

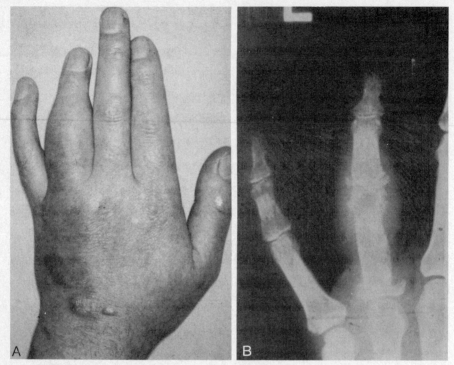

Figure 10–4. *A,* Chronic skin lesion. *B,* Associated punched-out bone cyst.

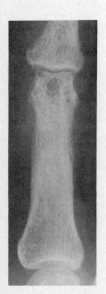

Figure 10–5. Early lytic lesion in head of proximal phalanx. There is "tunnelling" of the cortex under the periosteum.

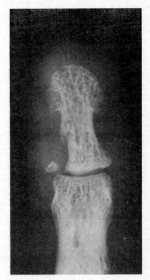

Figure 10–6. Lytic lesion at base of distal phalanx causing secondary joint damage. There is sequestrum formation but no periosteal reaction.

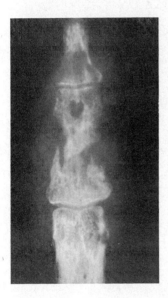

Figure 10–7. Rapidly advancing bone involvement with multiple fractures.

Figure 10–8. New cortex formation around lytic area in phalangeal head after 12 years. Permeative changes became sclerotic, and a pathological fracture in base of phalanx has healed.

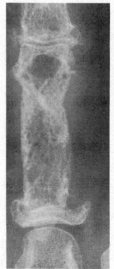
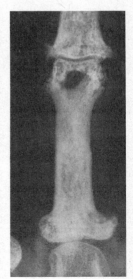

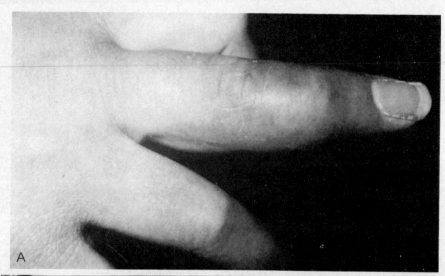

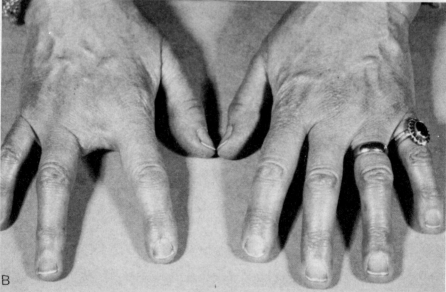

Figure 10–9. *A* and *B*, Sarcoid dactylitis. The finger was removed because it was considered to be tuberculous dactylitis.

absent even when cortical defects have been present for many years. In all three patients with destructive lesions, there were also lytic and permeative lesions, in one instance in the same bone.

Healing

Lytic lesions become corticated, forming the classical bone "cysts," permeative lesions regress so that a thick abnormal cortex reforms and becomes differentiated from medulla, and pathological fractures may unite without callus formation. The architecture may improve, but we have never seen a return to a completely normal bone. Although steroids often provide considerable symptomatic relief and even contribute to healing, this is not always so; one patient developed a permeative lesion while taking oral steroids for lupus pernio. The association of bone sarcoidosis with chronic skin lesions is again underlined, as nearly three-fourths of our patients had this combination. Lupus pernio has a very high incidence, and it is apparent that radiography of the hands and feet of patients with sarcoidosis is only worthwhile when chronic skin lesions are present (see Chapter 7). The course of bone sarcoidosis is slow and indolent in the patients with permeative lytic lesions, although the progression of the disease may be more rapid. There may be an apparent improvement of radiographical appearance with a return to tubular structure, but normality is never achieved and quiescence can never be guaranteed. Patients with bone sarcoidosis usually have chronic fibrotic sarcoidosis in other sites such as lungs, skin, and eyes. When bone involvement exists, the prognosis should be guarded, as we have shown a mortality of 21 per cent, four times greater than the overall mortality due to sarcoidosis.

JOINT INVOLVEMENT

By far the commonest clinical involvement, around 40 per cent,[21] is the polyarthralgia preceding or associated with erythema nodosum and bilateral hilar lymphadenopathy. It probably reflects a circulating immune complex (see p. 178). Far less common is the joint involvement secondary to bone sarcoidosis, and even less frequent is the chronic joint sarcoidosis with granulomatous involvement of a thickened synovium and joint effusion.[22] We have seen this rare manifestation in finger, knee, and elbow. These three types of joint involvement are brought into focus when they are classified into the categories of acute or chronic sarcoidosis. Flitting polyarthralgia associated with erythema nodosum is a feature of acute self-limiting sarcoidosis (Table 10–3). Joint involvement secondary to bone sarcoidosis and joint involvement with synovial thickening and effusion are both manifestations of chronic fibrotic sarcoidosis.

Table 10–3. Comparison of Acute Rheumatism with Arthralgia Preceding Erythema Nodosum

	Acute Rheumatism		Arthralgia Preceding Erythema Nodosum
Distribution of flitting pains			
Fever		Similar	
Sweating			
Cardiac murmur	Present		Absent
Rheumatic nodules	May be present		Absent
ESR	+	Very high	+
ECG	Abnormal		Normal
Anti-streptolysin titre	Elevated		Normal
Response to salicylates	Good		Indifferent

DACTYLITIS

Formerly, dactylitis was frequently due to tuberculosis. It is now more commonly associated with lupus pernio. The finger (or fingers) is swollen, painful to move, and slightly tender, and an x-ray will reveal a bone cyst. Treatment with steroids and weekly methotrexate doses provides symptomatic relief and may prevent deformity and contracture.

REFERENCES

1. Douglas AC, Macleod JG, Mathews JD. Symptomatic sarcoidosis of skeletal muscle. J Neurol Neurosurg Psychiat. 36:1034, 1973.
2. Stjernberg N, Cajander S, Truedsson H, Uddenfeldt P. Muscle involvement in sarcoidosis. Acta Med Scand. 209:213, 1981.
3. Lynch PG, Beansal DV: Granulomatous polymyositis. J Neurol Sci. 18:1, 1973.
4. Hinterbuchner CN, Hinterbuchner LP. Myopathic syndrome in muscular sarcoidosis. Brain. 87:355, 1964.
5. Dyken PR. Sarcoidosis of skeletal muscle. Neurology. 12:643, 1962.
6. Crompton MR, MacDermot V. Sarcoidosis associated with progressive muscular wasting and weakness. Brain 84:62, 1961.
7. Silverstein A, Siltzbach LE. Muscle involvement in sarcoidosis. Arch Neurol. 21:235, 1969.
8. Kreibich K. Uber lupus pernio. Arch Derm Syph (Wein). 71:3, 1904.
9. Schaumann J. Etudes histologiques et bacteriologique sur les manifestations medullaines du lymphogranuloma benin. Ann Derm Symph (Paris). 7:385, 1919.
10. Jungling O. Osteitis tuberculosa multiplex cystica. Forschner Rontgenstr. 27:375, 1920.
11. Besnier E: Lupus pernio de la face. Ann Derm Syph (Paris). 10:333, 1892.
12. James DG: Dermatological aspects of sarcoidosis. Quart J Med N S. 28:109, 1959.
13. Tervonen S, Karjalainen P, Valta R. Bone mineral in sarcoidosis. Acta Med Sand. 196:497, 1974.
14. Maycock RL, Bertrand P, Morrison CE, Scott JH. Manifestations of sarcoidosis: analysis of 145 patients with review of nine series selected from literature. Am J Med. 35:67, 1963.
15. Bouvier ME, Jejeune E, Quenseau P, Ryan M. Sarcoidosis avec lacunes cranieres. Rev Rheum. 39:205, 1972.

16. Curtis GT: Sarcoidosis of the nasal bones. Br J Radiol. 37:68, 1964.
17. Stein GN, Israel HL, Sones M. Roentgenographic study of skeletal lesions in sarcoidosis. Arch Intern Med. 97:532, 1956.
18. Turek SL. Sarcoid disease of bone at the ankle joint. J Bone Joint Surg. 35:465, 1953.
19. Berk RN, Brower TD. Vertebral sarcoidosis. Radiology. 82:600, 1964.
20. Young DA, Lamam NL. Sarcoidosis in the ribs. Am J Roentgenol. 114:553, 1972.
21. James DG, Neville E, Carstairs LS. Bone and joint sarcoidosis. Semin Arth Rheum. 1:53, 1976.
22. Scott DGI, Porto LOR, Lovell CR, Thomas GO. Chronic sarcoid synovitis in the Caucasian: an arthroscopic and histological study. Ann Rheumat Dis 40:121, 1981.
23. James DG, Neville E, Siltzbach LE, et al. A worldwide review of sarcoidosis. Ann NY Acad Sci. 278:321, 1976.

11

Miscellaneous Involvement

ALIMENTARY TRACT

Sarcoidosis only rarely affects the alimentary tract and is usually asymptomatic. However, granulomas are not uncommon and may be a feature of other systemic diseases of known and unknown causes or may simply appear as a reaction to a local cause. We therefore have to exclude the many causes of granulomas before accepting a diagnosis of sarcoidosis (Table 11–1).

Liver

The increasing use of needle biopsies of the liver in the investigation of primary liver disease and in diagnostic problems such as pyrexia of unknown cause frequently demonstrates unsuspected granulomas. The histology often reveals no causative agent, so that the onus of diagnosis is transferred to the clinician to sift collateral clinicoradiological evidence for the true explanation.

Klatskin reported on a large series of 565 patients with liver granulomas and found that the commonest causes in decreasing order of frequency were sarcoidosis, 217 cases (38 per cent); underlying liver disease, 174 (31 per cent); tuberculosis, 70 (12 per cent); and schistosomiasis, 19 (3 per cent).[1] These figures are very similar to those of our London series, in which 138 patients with liver granulomas were found to have sarcoidosis in 75 instances (54 per cent); primary biliary cirrhosis in 25 (19 per cent); miscellaneous recognisable disorders in 23 (17 per cent); and undiagnosed ailments in 14 (10 per cent) (Table 11–2). The Kveim-Siltzbach test is of value, for it is positive in about 70 per cent of patients with sarcoidosis and consistently negative in hepatic granulomas due to other causes.

Granulomas in sarcoidosis are usually isolated, randomly distributed, and often within portal tracts. As they are microscopic focal lesions, the residual scarring does not produce the diffuse fibrosis and nodular regeneration of cirrhosis and they rarely give rise to symptoms.

Intrahepatic cholestasis is a rare event, present in less than 1 per cent of patients in our series.[3] It is most frequent in black males, age 20 to 50 years, with jaundice, pruritus, hepatosplenomegaly, portal hypertension,

144

Table 11–1. Granulomas of the Alimentary Tract

Infections	Diseases of Unknown Cause
Tuberculosis	Sarcoidosis
Brucellosis	Primary biliary cirrhosis
Schistosomiasis	Granulomatous hepatitis
Histoplasmosis	Granulomatous gastritis
Blastomycosis	Crohn's disease
Coccidioidomycosis	Whipple's disease
Toxocara	**Reticulosis**
Q fever	Hodgkin's disease
Helminthiasis	Carcinoma
	Foreign Body Granulomas
	Drugs

and evidence of sarcoidosis in the lungs or eyes. There is a raised serum bilirubin level, increased IgG and SACE levels, positive Kveim-Siltzbach test, and negative serum mitochondrial antibodies. The granulomas are abundant and well formed with inconspicuous bile duct damage. Intrahepatic cholestasis is quite different from primary biliary cirrhosis, in which the hepatic granulomas are few and poor and bile ducts are seen to be damaged.

Sarcoid cholestasis persists for 20 years or so. It is nearly always associated with portal hypertension due to sarcoidosis.

Sarcoid Portal Hypertension

Sarcoid granulomas may involve the minute portal venous channels with cellular infiltration and narrowing of the sinusoids, leading to fibrosis and presinusoid portal hypertension. Wedged hepatic vein pressure is normal and less than that in the main portal vein.

Table 11–2. A Comparison of Hepatic Granulomas Investigated at Yale and London

Cause	Yale* No.	Yale* %	London† No.	London† %
Causes				
Sarcoidosis	217		75	
Liver disease	174	85	41	88
Tuberculosis	70		3	
Schistosomiasis	19		1	
Undiagnosed	37	7	14	10
Positive Kveim test	109	69	95	72
Total	565	100	138	100

*Data from Klatskin G. Hepatic granulomata: Problems in interpretation. Ann N Y Acad Sci. 278:427, 1976.

†Data from Neville E, Pyasena KHG, James DG. Granulomas of the liver. Postgrad Med J. 51:361, 1975.

Haemorrhage due to portal hypertension may develop early in its course, before a true nodular cirrhosis is present. If surgery is necessary to prevent fatal haemorrhage, then a porto-caval shunt should be considered. Good hepatocellular function allows for good surgical results without complicating portal-systemic encephalopathy.

Differential Diagnosis of Liver Granulomas

Infections

As elsewhere, tuberculosis must be excluded; this is often difficult because bacilli are only seen in about 10 per cent of otherwise proven cases. Do not forget that BCG vaccination is a frequent cause of liver granulomas.

Schistosomiasis must not be overlooked in endemic areas. The ova are usually readily recognised, and eosinophils may be prominent. Likewise in endemic areas, the necrosis seen with brucellosis, histoplasmosis, blasto-mycosis, coccidioidomycosis, toxocara, and Q fever is surrounded by eosin-ophilic necrosis, producing a halo effect.

Primary Liver Disease

The chief of these is primary biliary cirrhosis (PBC). There are several features that aid in distinguishing PBC from sarcoidosis (Table 11–3). We would emphasize that PBC predominates in women, pruritus is a prominent symptom, mitochondrial antibodies are present in nearly all cases, and disordered liver function is usual. The granulomas are clearly related to bile ducts, with consequent disruption of liver architecture and subsequent cirrhosis (Fig. 11–1).

Occasionally, incidental asymptomatic granulomas occur outside the liver, in portal lymph nodes, and even in the lung.[4] Rarely pulmonary symptoms may be prominent, suggesting an overlap syndrome.[5] Four such cases have been recently reported with radiological changes in the lung fields but no BHL; three showed pulmonary granulomas and all showed liver granulomas and changes of PBC.[6] Mitochondrial antibodies were strongly positive in all four, and the Kveim-Siltzbach test was negative in two and positive in one of three tested.

We consider PBC and sarcoidosis as separate entities, but as both may be related to circulating immune complexes,[7] overlap cases will occur.

After excluding liver granulomas of known cause and those associated with defined syndromes, such as sarcoidosis and PBC, we are left with what is sometimes referred to as "hepatic granulomas or granulomatous hepati-tis."[8] We prefer the former term because biopsies do not show hepatitis. These patients are often middle-aged men with fever and a disease confined

Table 11–3. A Comparison of Sarcoidosis and Primary Biliary Cirrhosis

	Features	Sarcoidosis	Primary Biliary Cirrhosis
Clinical	Sex F:M	Equal	8:1
	Decade of onset	30 and 40	50
	Erythema nodosum	Yes	No
	Uveitis	Yes	No
	Respiratory involvement	Yes	No
	Pruritus	No	Yes, eventually
	Jaundice	No	Yes, late
	Xanthomas	No	Yes, late
	Clubbing	No	Yes
	Hepatomegaly	Infrequently	Usually
	Splenomegaly	Yes	Yes
	Skin pigmentation	No	Yes
	Steatorrhoea	No	Yes, with jaundice
Radiology	Bilateral hilar lymphadenopathy	Yes	No
Immunology	Kveim-Siltzbach test	Positive in 80%	Always negative
	Depression of delayed-type hypersensitivity	Yes	Yes
	K:NK activity	Increased	Decreased
	OKT4:OHT8 lymphocyte ratio	Decrease in blood Increase in BAL	Decreased in blood
	Humoral immunity	Hyper-reactive	Hyper-reactive
	Immune complexes	Frequent	Frequent
	Mitochondrial antibodies	No	Yes (in 99%)
Biochemical	Calcium metabolism	Hypercalcaemia	Hypocalcaemia (steatorrhoea)
	Vitamin D	Sensitivity to	Lack of
	Raised		
	Alkaline phosphatase	Yes, minority	Yes, majority
	Serum cholesterol	No	Yes, majority
	Angiotensin-converting enzyme	Yes (in 60%)	Yes in up to 10%
Histology	Liver granulomas	Yes	Yes
Treatment	Corticosteroids	Helpful	Contraindicated
	Vitamin D	Contraindicated	Helpful
	Cholestyramine	Not necessary	Helpful
Prognosis		Good	Variable

to the liver. The Kveim-Siltzbach test is negative, but SACE may be elevated. Symptoms and fever may be halted by treatment with oral steroids, colchicine, and indomethacin.

Hepatic granulomas associated with Hodgkin's disease are important to recognise, as the consequences of mismanagement can be catastrophic. The granulomas are rich in eosinophils and usually unrelated to local tumour, which may be present in other organs.[9] The authors have seen one patient presenting with unexplained fever and eosinophil-rich liver granulomas with no evidence of tumour, which only become apparent one year later in cervical lymph nodes.

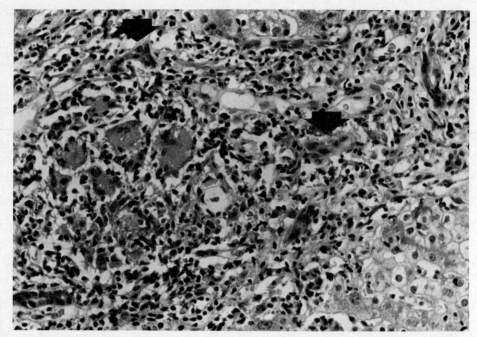

Figure 11–1. Primary biliary cirrhosis (arrows). Bile ducts surrounded by granulomas. H & E × 128.

Hepatic granulomas associated with acute inflammation of portal tracts, pericholangitis, may be induced by a number of drugs,[10, 11] including phenylbutazone, hydralazine, allopurinol, quinidine, methyldopa, diazepam, penicillin, sulphonamides, sulphonylurea, halothane, and carbamazepine.

Management

The management depends on the cause, so investigation must be thorough. Liver histology should be supplemented whenever possible by histology in other tissues. Radiology and bacteriology may also be helpful. There are a variety of treatments, depending on the cause (Table 11–4).

The significance of a granulomatous reaction may depend on the age of the patient (see Table 15–4) or on the region of the world in which it is detected (see Table 15–5).

The most useful tests for defining hepatic granulomas due to sarcoidosis are the chest radiograph, the Kveim-Siltzbach skin test, and the serum angiotensin-converting enzyme level.

Parotid Gland

Thirty-three of 537 (6 per cent) patients personally examined had parotid gland enlargement[12] (Fig. 11–2). It was bilateral in 24 (73 per cent), right-

Table 11–4. Management of Some Alimentary Tract Granulomas

Cause	Site	Helpful Investigations (Other Than Histology)	Treatment
Sarcoidosis	All tissues except pancreas and adrenals	Chest x-ray Siltzbach-Kveim test Slit lamp examination of eyes Serum calcium Urinary calcium Serum angiotensin-converting enzyme	Corticosteroids Oxyphenbutazone Chloroquine Potaba (?) Methotrexate Indomethacin
Primary biliary cirrhosis	Liver Spleen Lymph nodes	Serum mitochondrial antibodies Serum cholesterol Alkaline phosphatase Liver copper	Parenteral replacement of vitamins Calcium Cholestyramine Penicillamine Cyclosporin A
Tuberculosis	Liver, spleen Adrenals Intestine Peritoneum	Strongly positive tuberculin test Isolate organism	Isoniazid Rifampicin Ethambutol Streptomycin
Hodgkin's disease	Liver Spleen Intestine Lymph nodes	Abdominal CAT scan Lymphangiography Splenectomy	Quadruple chemotherapy Radiotherapy
Crohn's regional ileitis	Intestine Liver Perineum	Radiography	Azathioprine Salazopyrine Metronidazole
Brucellosis	Liver Spleen	Occupation exposure Skin test Serum antibodies	Tetracycline
Toxocara infestation	Liver Lungs Brain	Skin test Eosinophilia Examine fundi	Thiabendazole
Febrile hepatic granulomas	Liver Spleen	Exclusion of all else	Steroids Colchicine Indomethacin

sided in 6, and left-sided in 3 patients. It was slightly more common in women, who presented in three-fourths of instances in the 20- to 40-year age group. There was widespread involvement of other systems (Table 11–5). Uveoparotitis (Heerfordt's syndrome) was noted in 19 patients, and in 5 instances there was concomitant facial nerve palsy. The fact that Bell's palsy was so infrequent suggests that it is not due to pressure from the enlarged parotid gland.

The course of involvement of the parotid gland and that of the intra-thoracic tract mirrored each other and were of two types. In 16 patients there was spontaneous resolution within six months. In the remainder steroid therapy was necessary; in these patients the response was grudging, slow, and incomplete. Thus, parotid gland enlargement may be either acute, transient, and self-limiting, or it may be chronic and persistent.

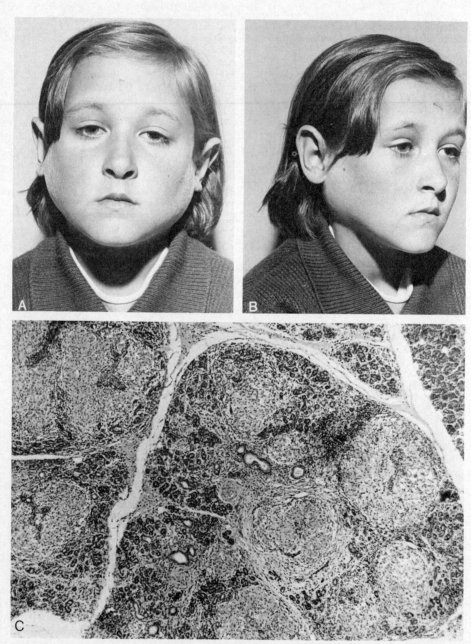

Figure 11–2. Parotid gland enlargement due to sarcoidosis. *A* and *B*, Clinical presentation. *C*, Histological specimen. H & E × 80.

Table 11–5. Features of 33 Patients with Parotid Gland Enlargement
Due to Sarcoidosis

Feature	Patients	
	No.	%
Number in whole series	33/537	6
Female	21	63
Bilateral	24	73
Age at Onset (years)		
1–20	1	
21–30	12 ⎫ 25	75
31–40	13 ⎭	
41	6	
Involvement of		
Intrathoracic	28	84
Peripheral lymphadenopathy	19	58
Skin	15	46
Spleen	9	27
Uveal tract	19	58
Lacrimal glands	8	24
Facial nerve	5	15
Skin Tests		
Positive Kveim	10/13	77
Negative tuberculin	17/21	81
Abnormal Serum Globulins	10/20	50

Mouth

The minor salivary glands and gums are biopsy sources and are helpful in confirming the diagnosis of sarcoidosis (see Chapter 3). Localised sarcoid tissue reactions to mucous gland cysts must not be misconstrued as sarcoidosis, for involvement of oral mucosa is rare in sarcoidosis.[13]

Granulomatous Cheilitis (Melkersson-Rosenthal Syndrome)

This rare disorder involves the mouth and adjacent tissues (Fig. 11–3; see also color plate 6). There is granulomatous involvement of the oral

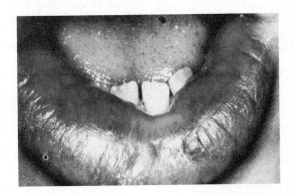

Figure 11–3. Swollen indurated lower lip (with granulomas) in a patient with Melkersson-Rosenthal syndrome.

mucosa, gum, lips, tongue, pharynx, eyelids, and skin of the face. In 1928, Melkersson first described an association between facial oedema and facial paralysis.[14] Rosenthal added lingua plicata, or scrotal tongue, to the clinical picture.[15] Other variations include oedema of the gums and scalp, salivary gland dysfunction, granulomatous blepharitis, trigeminal neuralgia, Raynaud's phenomenon, and even chronic hypertrophic granulomatous vulvitis.

The cause is unknown, but granulomatous cheilitis can be kept under satisfactory control by intermittent courses of steroids or a combination of steroids and azathioprine.

Granulomatous cheilitis is mistaken for sarcoidosis when an otherwise fit adult develops facial nerve palsy, swollen eyelids, and salivary gland dysfunction and a biopsy of the involved area reveals sarcoid tissue. Other features of sarcoidosis, such as uveitis, chest x-ray changes, and a positive Kveim test, are either absent or negative.

Stomach

Stomach involvement in sarcoidosis is very rare, is usually incidental and symptomless, and is only exceptionally of clinical importance. The differential diagnosis includes primary intestinal diseases, in particular Crohn's disease, the rare isolated granulomatous gastritis, and local isolated granulomas, which frequently are related to benign or malignant ulceration. Tuberculosis is now a rare cause of gastric granulomas.

With increasing use of endoscopy the incidence of symptomless granulomas in sarcoid patients is an appreciable 11 per cent,[16] although in a large autopsy series (30 cases) none were found.[17] The granulomas are often single and are mainly found in the mucosa.

Symptomatic sarcoidosis of the stomach is distinguished by a large number of granulomas distributed throughout the wall with a curious predilection for the distal, pyloric end. Such cases may present with pyloric obstruction and may even mimic diffuse carcinoma of the stomach (linitis plastica).[18] However, it is difficult to accept many of the single case reports as examples of sarcoidosis, as the lesions were often confined to the stomach, with sometimes local involvement of adjacent glands or spleen or both.[19]

Similar cases have been labelled Crohn's disease[20] or isolated granulomatous gastritis,[21, 22] both of which are easily confused with sarcoidosis in affecting predominantly the pyloric region with numerous granulomas throughout the full thickness, also mimicking diffuse carcinoma. Gastric Crohn's disease is distinguished by the frequent involvement of other parts of the intestine, notably the duodenum and jejunum, and the absence of disease in other systems. Isolated granulomatous gastritis is considered to be a separate entity, occurring most commonly in older subjects and unassociated with either multisystem involvement or involvement of other parts of the gastro-intestinal tract.

Twelve cases of sarcoid granulomas associated with gastric ulceration, five pre-operatively diagnosed as benign and seven pre-operatively diagnosed as carcinoma, have been recorded in Japan. These were presumably all local reactions, as none had BHL, although interestingly seven patients were tuberculin negative and five were Kveim positive.[23] The authors have seen a patient with ulcerating gastric carcinoma whose greater curve glands, but not the tumour, were grossly enlarged and replaced by sarcoid granulomas but with no other system involved.

Oesophageal involvement in sarcoidosis is exceptional, as only one case has been recorded.[24]

Intestine

Crohn's Disease

Intestinal involvement in sarcoidosis is extremely rare, and most reports are probably examples of Crohn's disease, a condition practically confined to the intestinal tract and with many features distinguishing it from sarcoidosis (Table 11–6). We would emphasize that in Crohn's disease, granulomas are only present in around one-half of the cases,[25] the Kveim-Siltzbach test is negative,[26] and SACE levels are within normal limits.[27]

There are a few reports of patients with both diseases occurring either at the same time or sequentially[28, 29] but no evidence to suggest a common cause.

Table 11–6. Comparison of Sarcoidosis and Crohn's Disease

	Features	Sarcoidosis	Crohn's Disease
Clinical	Sex F:M	Equal	Equal
	Decade of onset	30 and 40	30 and 60
	Erythema nodosum	Yes	Yes
	Other skin lesions	Yes (25%)	Mucocutaneous, often ulcerative
	Respiratory involvement	Yes	No
	Intestinal involvement	No	Yes
	Ocular involvement	Yes (25%)	No
	Malabsorption	No	Yes
	Peritonitis	No	Common
	Ankylosing spondylitis	No	Yes
Radiology	Chest	Abnormal	Normal
	Barium	Normal	Abnormal
Immunology	Kveim-Siltzbach test	Positive (80%)	Always negative
	Depression-delayed hypersensitivity	Yes	Yes
	Humoral immunity	Hyper-reactive	Hyper-reactive
Biochemical	Calcium metabolism	Often hypercalcaemic	Hypocalcaemic
Histology	Intestinal granulomas	Very rare	50%, confined to gut
Treatment	Surgery	Never	Yes
	Corticosteroids	Helpful	Helpful

Localised Granulomas

Localised granulomas of the alimentary tract may be a reaction to foreign material such as faecal debris, mucins, and fats, as in cholecystitis, cystica glandularis, diverticulitis, and, rarely, ulcerative colitis. They are identified by the finding of the inciting agent and foreign body rather than Langhans giant cells and sometimes eosinophils.[30]

The localised granulomatous nodules resulting from a reaction to Biosorb starch glove powder are well recognised[31] (Fig. 11–4). The presence of Maltese cross, birefringent, rounded (around 12 μ in diameter), PAS-positive starch granules within macrophages and the numerous and epithelioid-like foreign body giant cells easily distinguishes the lesions from sarcoidosis. More recently it has been shown that the reaction is not just a foreign body response but an immunological one. Affected patients show a delayed hypersensitivity reaction to intradermal starch suspensions and, after about 10 days, a histological granulomatous reaction. Having abandoned talc in surgical gloves and other starch materials, we still have a problem. Similar peritoneal granulomas may also occur from other starches, such as potatoes, following intestinal perforation.[33]

Talc granulomas are well recognised if sections are examined with polarised light, which shows up brilliant birefringent, silicate crystals (Fig. 11–5).

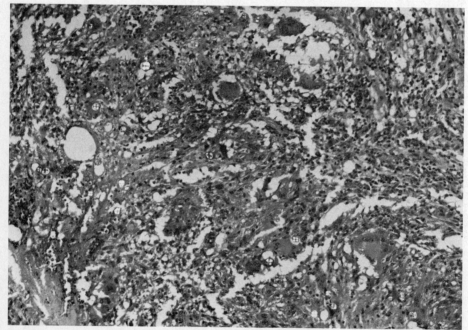

Figure 11–4. Peritoneal Biosorb starch granuloma. Note Maltese cross granules. H & E (polarised) × 128.

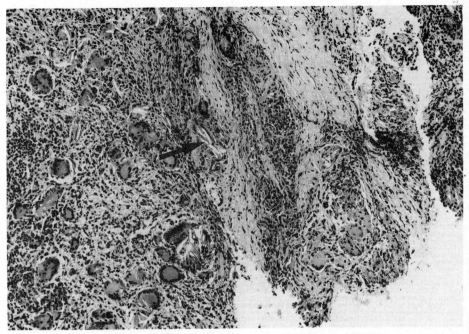

Figure 11–5. Peritoneal talc granuloma (arrow). H & E (polarised) × 150.

Whipple's Disease

This is not a common disease, but it does cause widespread alimentary tract granulomas, including hepatic granulomas. It has been confused with both sarcoidosis (Table 11–7) and Crohn's regional enteritis. The management of each is different, so it is important to recognise the differences. Think of Whipple's disease when the older patient has steatorrhoea and widespread alimentary tract granulomas. At first the patient is suspected of having tuberculosis or a reticulosis, but, in due course, the benign behaviour of the disease suggests sarcoidosis. Intestinal biopsy with the appropriate staining is definitive, disclosing foamy histiocytes that are PAS-positive (Fig. 11–6).

CHILDHOOD

Sarcoidosis is rarely a paediatric problem. In our initial series of 537 patients, it presented in only one child under 10 years of age and only in 25 (5 per cent) under 20 years of age. In a review of 3,000 cases from the world literature, just under 4 per cent of patients were less than 15 years of age.[34] Symptomatic sarcoidosis is uncommon in childhood, but asymptomatic disease is increasingly recognised in some countries.[35, 36]

Table 11–7. Differential Diagnosis of Sarcoidosis and Whipple's Disease

Feature	Sarcoidosis	Whipple's Disease
Other names		Lipophagic intestinal granulomatosis
Sex	Equal	Males predominate
Decade of onset	30 and 40	40 through 70
Non-deforming arthritis	Yes with erythema nodosum	Characteristic initial feature
Steatorrhoea	No	Severe principal feature
Diarrhoea	No	Yes
Weight loss	Infrequent	Frequent
Lymphadenopathy	27%	40%
Polyserositis	No	Yes
PAS stain of macrophages in lymph node	Negative	Positive
Jejunal biopsy	Normal	Villous atrophy
Electron microscopy	Negative	Bacilliform bodies
Treatment	Corticosteroids	Antibiotics

In the US,[37] children between the ages of 8 and 15 develop multisystem disease with involvement of the lungs, lymph nodes, and eyes, as in adults. The picture in children 4 years and younger is different.[38] This young child usually presents with a rash, arthritis, and uveitis without demonstrable pulmonary disease. The American child is most likely to be black and symptomatic with a high incidence of reticulo-endothelial involvement, hyperglobulinaemia, and hypercalcaemia.

By way of contrast,[37] the Japanese or Hungarian[36] child with sarcoidosis is detected by routine chest radiography, is usually symptom-free, and shows few abnormal physical signs. In a recent series of 23 patients in France,[39] 70 per cent were asymptomatic and six were recognised by routine chest radiography.

What can we learn from a more detailed comparison of patients in the US, Japan, Hungary, and France (Table 11–8)?

Race and Sex. As with black adults, black children are more likely to show severe and extensive disease than Caucasian and Japanese children. Of those patients in the US series, 72 per cent were blacks; there were 2 black patients out of 23 in the French series. The sex incidence was broadly similar in all four series.

Symptoms. In both the US (87 per cent) and France (76 per cent), the majority of patients presented with or developed symptoms, compared with only 7 per cent in Japan and 16 per cent in Hungary. This important difference is explained by the detection of Japanese and Hungarian cases by routine chest radiography of school children. Such practice may reveal a very high incidence of asymptomatic disease. In one middle grade school in Sendai, Japan, the incidence was 5.9/10,000 children with an overall rate of 1/10,000. It is interesting to speculate the results of similar investigations in the US and the United Kingdom.

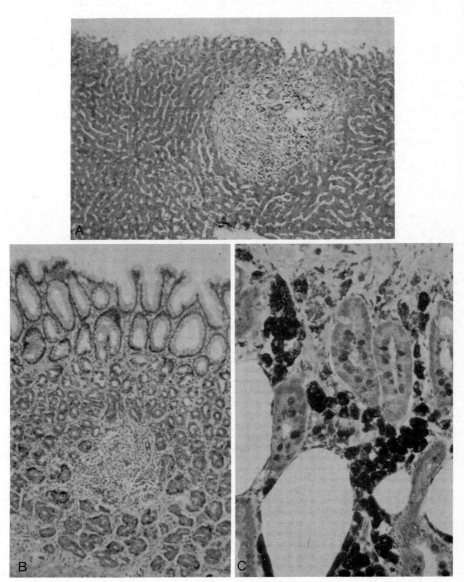

Figure 11–6. Whipple's disease. *A*, Non-specific liver granuloma. H & E × 60. *B*, Non-specific granuloma in intestine. H & E × 80. *C*, PAS -positive macrophages. PAS × 200.

Table 11–8. Childhood Sarcoidosis (Under 15 Years of Age)

Features	US* No.	%	Japan* No.	%	Hungary† No.	%	France‡ No.	%
Number of patients	40	100	45	100	31	100	23	100
Race	29	72(black)	Japanese		Caucasian		2	(black— 8%)
Male	19	47	27	60	17	55	13	56
Symptomatic	35	87	3	7	5	16	17	74
Histology								
Tissue	40	100	40	88	30	99	21	90
Kveim	0	0	4	10	0	0	6/8	75
Hilar lymphadenopathy								
Bilateral (Stage III)	40	100	44	98	22	75	0	0
Bilateral + lung (Stage II)	0	0	0	0	8	25	18	80
Unilateral	0	0	0	0	2	0	0	0
Extrathoracic lesions								
Peripheral adenopathy	30	67	18	40			7	30
Hepatomegaly	12	30	0	0			Not specified	
Splenomegaly	9	23	0	0	Not specified		Not specified	
Ocular	9	23	6	13			9	40
Bone cysts	4	10	6	13			Not specified	
Skin								
EN	0	0	0	0	3	1	0	0
Other	10	25	0	0	Not specified		7	30
Hyperglobulinaemia	24	36	11/43	26	Infrequent		9	40
Hypercalcaemia	7	33	2/37	5	2	6	6	26
Prognosis								
Remission (with or without steroids)	35	87	38	88	Not specified		21	90
Progression	5	13	1	2			2	9
Blindness	2	5	1	2			2	9
Pulmonary fibrosis	3	0	0	0			0	0

*Data from Kendig EL, Niitu Y. Sarcoidosis in Japanese and American children: a comparison. *In* Jones Williams W, Davies BH (eds): Sarcoidosis. Cardiff, Alpha and Omega Press. p 572, 1980.

†Data from Loos T. Sarcoidosis in children. *In* Djuric B (ed): Proc 3rd Internat Conf Sarcoidosis. Yugoslavia, New Faculty, Novi Sad. p 335, 1982.

‡Data from Baculard A, Couvreur J, Tournier G, Gernaux J. Sarcoidosis in children, an epidemiological and clinical approach. *In* Chretien J, Marsac J, Saltiel JC (eds): Proc 9th Internat Conf Sarcoidosis. Paris, Pergamon Press. p 621, 1983.

Chest Involvement. In the US and Japan all patients were radiographical Stage I. One-fourth of the Hungarian patients had Stage II disease, and there was a very high incidence (80 per cent) of Stage II disease in France. The two Hungarian patients with unilateral hilar lymphadenopathy appear to be unique.

Extrathoracic Lesions. Peripheral lymphadenopathy was common in American children (67 per cent) and frequent in Japanese (40 per cent) and French children (30 per cent) but not reported in Hungarian children. Hepatomegaly (30 per cent) and splenomegaly (23 per cent) were only observed in the American children. The generalised involvement of the reticulo-endothelial system is considerably more common in children (particularly American children) than in adult patients (see Table 4–1). Peripheral lymphadenopathy is unusual (27 per cent), and hepatomegaly (10 per cent) and splenomegaly (12 per cent) are even less frequent among adults (see Table 4–1).

Eye involvement was common in the French series (40 per cent) and was found in 23 per cent of American children. Although the Japanese cases were mainly asymptomatic, eye involvement was not uncommon (13 per cent), and one patient became blind.

Interestingly, erythema nodosum was only reported in Hungarian patients (3 of 31 cases). Other skin lesions were reported in 25 per cent of American children and occasionally in French children (number not specified). As in adults, such cases show more extensive disease and a more protracted course.

Prognosis. Although the majority of children (90 per cent) recover with or without steroid therapy, as with adults a few develop blindness and pulmonary fibrosis. We do not know why some children fare far worse than others. Could it be ethnic differences or HLA affinities or both? Could there be an impoverished sarcoid soil under which circumstances the disease becomes chronic, fibrotic, or complicated?

Polyarthropathy in Children

Polyarthropathy in children is rare and most frequently presents in those under the age of 5 years.[40] It may be difficult to diagnose, as hilar lymphadenopathy and pulmonary changes are absent or inconspicuous. Both constitutional and joint symptoms are minimal. The arthritis predominantly affects major joints, producing large boggy synovial proliferation and tendon sheath effusions. Synovial biopsies show classical sarcoid granulomas. Uveitis and salivary gland involvement are common, and skin lesions are persistent.

Polyarthropathy is usually distinguishable from the more common polyarticular juvenile rheumatoid arthritis (JRA), which is characterised by a later onset (5 to 15 years), marked constitutional symptoms, pauci-articular symptoms, and lymphocytic synovial infiltration. Uveitis may be common to both sarcoidosis and JRA, but the high incidence of antinuclear factors (88 per cent in JRA, absent in sarcoidosis) is of value in the differential diagnosis.[41] Serum angiotensin-converting enzyme is often raised in childhood sarcoidosis[42] but not recognised to be raised in JRA.

The very rare granulomatous vasculitis with polyarthropathy must also be distinguished from sarcoidosis; some cases are now recognised to be familial.[43, 44] The disease affects small joints. As in JRA, constitutional symptoms are marked. The granulomatous vasculitis affects both large and small vessels and is often associated with hypertension. The involvement of large vessels, the occasional extravascular granulomas, the absence of skin lesions, and the inherited pattern all serve to distinguish this group from polyarteritis. It is likely, however, that there are many overlap syndromes of "vascular" arthropathy, including systemic lupus erythematosus, scleroderma, and, in the elderly, giant cell arteritis.

PREGNANCY

As sarcoidosis is common in the child-bearing years, the usually favourable effect of pregnancy on the course of the disease is well recognised. This is normally attributed to the increased steroid output of pregnancy similar to that of patients on steroids; the dose can often be decreased or even stopped. There is no evidence that the foetus is ever affected, and normal delivery can be expected.

A recent report on the effect of 35 pregnancies on 18 patients showed no effect in 9 and clinical and radiological improvement in 6 patients.[45] A deleterious effect was noted in only three patients, all with chronic and extrathoracic disease.

KIDNEY

We were able to diagnose renal involvement during life in only 10 (1 per cent) patients, and another report cited 4.3 per cent.[46] Recent biopsy studies would suggest a more realistic incidence of 10 of 25 (40 per cent),[47] and necropsy studies also indicate a frequency of 13 to 39 per cent.[43, 49] The granulomas are usually sparse and randomly distributed in the cortex and medulla, although massive granulomatous infiltration may rarely occur.[50, 51] Granulomas may be silent and without evidence of renal dysfunction, or they may be associated with hypercalciuria[47] or immune complexes.[52] A number of non-granulomatous features may be found including varying amounts of non-specific round cell infiltration, pyelonephritis, hyalinisation of arterioles and glomeruli, and one instance of amyloidosis.[47] Many of these changes may be coincidental, although hypercalcaemia and nephrocalcinosis are causative factors. The association of glomerulonephritis with sarcoidosis, although uncommon, is increasingly recognised, and the majority are of membranous type.[53-55] A number of investigators have described an associated immune complex deposition.[53, 54, 57-59] Mikami emphasizes the importance of concurrent micro-angiopathy in other sites such as retina and muscle as evidence that multisystem immune complex deposition is part of the basic pathogenesis of sarcoidosis.[53]

Nephrocalcinosis is present in about 1 per cent of sarcoid patients, usually a late sequela of persistent abnormal calcium metabolism or calciferol therapy. It is a serious complication, as recurrent calculi lead to pyelonephritis, renal fibrosis, and consequent renal failure, which is little influenced by treatment.

REFERENCES

1. Klatskin G. Hepatic granulomata: Problems in interpretation. Ann NY Acad Sci. 278:427, 1976.
2. Neville E, Pyasena KHG, James DG. Granulomas of the liver. Postgrad Med J. 51:361, 1975.
3. Bass NM, Burroughs AK, Scheuer PJ, James DG, Sherlock S. Chronic intrahepatic cholestasis due to sarcoidosis. Gut. 23:417, 1982.
4. Fox RA, James DG, Scheuer PJ, Sharma O, Sherlock S. Impaired delayed hypersensitivity in primary biliary cirrhosis. Lancet. 1:959, 1969.
5. Maddrey WC, Johns CJ, Boitnott JK, Iber FL. Sarcoidosis and chronic hepatic disease: a clinical and pathological study of 20 patients. Medicine (Balt). 49:375, 1970.
6. Fagan EA, Moore-Gillon JC, Turner-Warwick M. Multiorgan granulomas and mitochondrial antibodies. N Engl J Med. 308:572, 1983.
7. Sherlock S, Thomas HC, Potter BJ, Jain S, Epstein O. Primary biliary cirrhosis as a granulomatous disease. *In* Jones Williams W, Davies BH (eds): Sarcoidosis. Cardiff, Alpha and Omega Press. p 746, 1980.
8. Simon HB, Wolff SM. Granulomatous hepatitis and prolonged fever of unknown origin: a study of 13 patients. Medicine. 52:1, 1973.
9. Jones Williams W, Jones DL, Whittacker JL. Isolated sarcoid-like granulomas in Hodgkin's disease. *In* Jones Williams W, Davies BH (eds): Sarcoidosis. Cardiff, Alpha and Omega Press. p 758, 1980.
10. Ishak KG, Kirchner JP, Dhar JK. Granulomas and cholestatic–hepatocellular injury associated with phenylbutazone. Report of two cases. Am J Dig Dis. 22:611, 1977.
11. Mitchell MC, Boitnott JK, Arregui A, Maddrey WC. Granulomatous hepatitis associated with carbamazepine therapy. Am J Med. 71:733, 1981.
12. Greenberg G, Anderson R, Sharpstone P, James DG. Enlargement of parotid gland due to sarcoidosis. Br Med J. 2:861, 1964.
13. Gold RS, Flanders NJ, Sager E. Oral sarcoidosis: review of the literature. J Oral Surg. 34(3):237, 1976.
14. Melkersson E. tt fall av recidiverande facialispares. i sam band med angioneurotiskt odem. Hygiea. 90:737, 1928.
15. Rosenthal C. Klinische-erbbiolog ischer beitrag für konstitution—pathologie: gemeinsames auftreten von (rezidivierender familiaiver). Facialislahmung, angioneurotischem gesichtsödem und lingua. Plicata in arthritismus—familien. Z Neurol Psychol. 131:475, 1931.
16. Palmer ED. A note on silent sarcoidosis of gastric mucosa. J Lab Clin Med. 52:231, 1968.
17. Longcope WT, Freiman DG. A study of sarcoidosis. Medicine. 31:1, 1952.
18. Orie NGM, Van Rijssel TG, Van der Zwaag ThG. Pyloric stenosis in sarcoidosis. Acta Med Scand. 138:141, 1950.
19. Scadding JG. Sarcoidosis. London, Eyre and Spottiswoode. p 321, 1967.
20. Pryse Davies J. Gastro-duodenal Crohn's disease. J Clin Pathol. 17:90, 1964.
21. Fahimi HD, Deren JJ, Gottlieb LS, Zamcheck N. Isolated granulomatous gastritis: its relationship to disseminated sarcoidosis and regional enteritis. Gastroenterology. 45:161, 1963.
22. Negus D. Giant cell granuloma of the stomach. Br J Surg. 53:475, 1966.
23. Tachibana T, Murato Y, Kitano K, Taketani H. Gastric sarcoidosis. *In* Iwai K, Hosoda Y (eds): Proc 6th Internat Conf Sarcoidosis. Tokyo, Univ of Tokyo Press. p 603, 1974.
24. Polachek AA, Matre WJ. Gastrointestinal sarcoidosis. Report of a case involving oesophagus. Am J Dig Dis. 9:429, 1964.
25. Jones Williams W. Histology of Crohn's syndrome. Gut. 5:510, 1964.
26. Siltzbach LE, Vieira LOBD, Topilsky M, Janowitz HD. Is there Kveim responsiveness in Crohn's disease? Lancet. ii:634, 1971.
27. Silverstein E, et al. Angiotensin-converting enzyme in Crohn's disease and ulcerative colitis. *In* Chretien J, Marsac J, Saltiel JC (eds): Proc 9th Internat Conf Sarcoidosis. Paris, Pergamon Press. p 572, 1983.
28. Dines DE, DeRemee RA, Green PA. Sarcoidosis associated with regional enteritis (Crohn's disease). Minnes Med. 54:617, 1971.
29. Padilla AJ, Sparberg M. Regional enteritis and sarcoidosis in one patient. Gastroenterology. 63:153, 1972.
30. Jones Williams W. Sarcoid-like granulomas of alimentary tract. *In* Turiaf J, Chabot J, James

DG, Zatouroff M (eds): La Sarkoidose. Rapp 4th Internat Conf Sarcoidosis. Paris, Masson & C. p 35, 1967.

31. Myers RN, Deaver JM, Brown CE. Granulomatous peritonitis due to starch glove powder: a clinical and experimental study. Ann Surg. 151:106, 1960.

32. Grant JBF, Davies JD, Espiner HJ, Eltringham WK. Diagnosis of granulomatous starch peritonitis by delayed hypersensitivity skin reactions. Br J Surg. 69:197, 1982.

33. Davies JD, Ansell ID. Food starch granulomatous peritonitis. J Clin Pathol. 36:435, 1983.

34. McGovern JP, Merritt DM. Sarcoidosis in childhood. Adv Paediatric. 8:97, 1956.

35. Niitu Y, Horikawa M, Suetake T, Hasegawa S, Kubota H, Komatsu S. Intrathoracic sarcoidosis in children. In Iwai K, Hosoda Y (eds): Proc 6th Internat Conf Sarcoidosis. Japan, Univ of Tokyo Press. p 507, 1974.

36. Loos T, Sarcoidosis in children. In Djuric B (ed): Proc 3rd European Conf Sarcoidosis. Yugoslavia, New Faculty, Novi Sad. p 335, 1982.

37. Kendig EL, Niitu Y. Sarcoidosis in Japanese and American children: a comparison. In Jones Williams W, Davies BH (eds): Proc 8th Internat Conf Sarcoidosis. Cardiff, Alpha and Omega Press. p 572, 1980.

38. Hetherington S. Sarcoidosis in young children. Am J Dis Children. 136:13, 1982.

39. Bacular A, Couvreur J, Tournier G, Gerneaux J. Sarcoidosis in children, an epidemiological and clinical approach. In Chretien J, Marsac J, Saltiel JC (eds): Proc 9th Internat Conf Sarcoidosis. Paris, Pergamon Press. p 621, 1983.

40. North AF, Fink CW, Gibson WM, Levson JE, Schuchter SL, Howard WK. Sarcoid arthritis in children. Am J Med. 48:449, 1970.

41. Schaller JG, Johnson GD, Holborrow EJ, Ansell BM, Smiley WK. The association of antinuclear antibodies with the chronic irridocyclitis of juvenile rheumatoid arthritis (Still's disease). Arthritis Rheum. 17:409, 1974.

42. Niitu Y, Nagayama H, Horikawa M. Angiotensin-converting enzyme activity in sarcoidosis in children. In Jones Williams W, Davies BH (eds): Sarcoidosis. Cardiff, Alpha and Omega Press. p 291, 1980.

43. Rotenstein D, Gibbas DL, Majmudar B, Chastain EA. Familial granulomatous arteritis with polyarthritis of juvenile onset. N Engl J Med. 306:86, 1982.

44. DiLiberti JH. Granulomatous vasculitis. N Engl J Med. 306:1365, 1982.

45. Agha FP, Yade A, Amendola MA, Cooper RF. Effects of pregnancy on sarcoidosis. Surg Gynaecol Obstet. 155:817, 1982.

46. Maycock RL, Bertrand P, Morrison CE, Scott JH. Manifestations of sarcoidosis: analysis of 145 patients with a review of nine series selected from the literature. Am J Med. 35:67, 1963.

47. Lebacq E, Verhaegen H. Renal involvement in sarcoidosis. In Levinsky L, Macholda F (eds): 5th Internat Conf Sarocidosis. Prague, Universita Karlova. p 323, 1971.

48. Longcope WT, Freiman DG. A study of sarcoidosis. Medicine. 31:1, 1952.

49. Huang CT, Heurich AE, Sutton AL, Rosen Y, Lyons HA. Mortality in sarcoidosis. In Jones Williams W, Davies BH (eds): Sarcoidosis. Cardiff, Alpha and Omega Press. p 522, 1980.

50. Berger KW, Relman AS. Renal impairment due to sarcoid infiltration of the kidneys: Report of a case proved by renal biopsies before and after treatment with cortisone. N Engl J Med. 252:45, 1955.

51. Ogilvie RI, Kaye M, Moore S. Granulomatous sarcoid disease of the kidney. Ann Internat Med. 61:711, 1964.

52. Fall WF. Nonhypercalcaemic sarcoid nephropathy. Arch Internat Med. 130:285, 1972.

53. Mikami R, Shibata S, Shimada Y, Fuse Y, Kobayashi F, Ryujiin Y. Microangiopathy and nephropathy in sarcoidosis. In Mikami R, Hosoda Y (eds): Sarcoidosis. Tokyo, Univ Tokyo Press. p 109, 1981.

54. Taylor RG, Fisher C, Hoffbrand BI. Sarcoidosis and membranous glomerulonephritis: a significant association. Br Med J. 284:1297, 1982.

55. McCoy RC, Tisher CC. Glomerulonephritis associated with sarcoidosis. Am J Pathol. 68:339, 1972.

56. Salomen MI, Tung PP, Kornad CH, Edward JK, Tchertkoff V. Membranous glomerulopathy in a patient with sarcoidosis. Arch Pathol. 99:479, 1975.

57. Yamagata Y, et al. A sarcoidosis case accompanying nephrotic syndromes. In Proc 9th Japan Conf on Renal Studies, West Chapter, April 1979.

58. Palestro G, Mazzuco G, Coda R. Granulonephritis and sarcoidosis. Report of a case. Panminerva Med. 17:127, 1975.

59. Briner J, Gartmann J. Glomerulonephritis bei Sarkoidose. Schweiz Med Wschr. 108:401, 1978.

12

Biochemistry

The majority of patients with sarcoidosis in our series have presented a number of biochemical abnormalities (Table 12–1).

Abnormal calcium metabolism is demonstrated in up to 40 per cent of the patients, but permanent renal damage due to nephrocalcinosis as a result of persistent derangement of calcium metabolism is rare. Raised immunoglobulin levels are commonplace; one-half of the Caucasians and two-thirds of the West Indians had elevated IgG levels. Abnormal immunoglobulin levels carry no obvious diagnostic or prognostic significance. Raised alkaline phosphatase levels reflect space-occupying hepatic granulomas or, rarely, skeletal involvement due to bone cysts. Serum angiotensin-converting enzyme (SACE) levels are elevated in 60 per cent of patients. The highest SACE activity is found in patients with severe parenchymal lung infiltration due to sarcoidosis and the lowest levels in those with inactive disease or after successful management with steroid drugs. SACE levels are not frequently elevated in patients with other granulomatous conditions—Crohn's disease, primary biliary cirrhosis, active tuberculosis, extrinsic allergic alveolitis, and tumours (Hodgkin's disease).

CALCIUM LEVELS

Hypercalcaemia and hypercalciuria are well-recognised biochemical features of sarcoidosis and have been noted in all racial groups. In a world survey, James and associates[1] noted hypercalcaemia in 200 of 1,760 (11 per cent) patients (Table 12–2).

In our London series, hypercalcaemia was found in 99 of 547 patients (18 per cent), taking an upper limit of normal of 10.5 mg (2.6 mmol/l), and hypercalciuria in 77 of 192 patients (40 per cent), taking an upper limit of urinary calcium excretion rate at 300 mg/24 hr (7.5 mmol/24 hr) (Table 12–1). It is interesting to note that abnormal calcium metabolism is less likely to occur in West Indian patients and is most likely to occur at two stages of the disease: in the 21- to 30-year age group when the disease is acute and in those over 41 years of age in whom troublesome chronic sarcoidosis occurs (Table 12–3). Residual irreversible renal damage due to nephrocalcinosis is described but in this series was rare, occurring in only 10 out of 818 patients.

163

Table 12–1. Biochemical Abnormalities in a Series of
818 Patients with Sarcoidosis

Blood Chemical	No. Patients	Abnormal* No.	%	Normal Range (at 37° C)
Albumin	526	82	16	36–52 gm/l
Globulin	526	161	31	20–34 gm/l
Calcium	547	99	18	2.2–2.6 mmol/l
Phosphate	343	47	13	0.8–1.4 mmol/l
Alkaline phosphatase	252	58	23	20–80 IU/l
Urea	213	42	20	2.5–7.0 mmol/l
Uric acid (urate)	50	9	18	0.1–0.42 mmol/l
Bilirubin	164	12	7	2–14 μmol/l

*Outside the normal range of values in our laboratory.

Table 12–2. Serum Globulin Estimation in 1,832 Patients
and Serum Calcium Levels in 1,760 Patients with
Sarcoidosis in a World Survey of Sarcoidosis*

	Globulins Patients Tested	Elevated No.	%	Calcium Patients Tested	Elevated No.	%
London	250	85	34	238	57	24
New York	260	158	61	236	33	14
Paris	212	48	23	249	17	7
Los Angeles	150	129	86	150	16	11
Tokyo	102	25	25	102	9	9
Reading	240	97	40	229	32	14
Lisbon	55	36	65	47	13	28
Edinburgh	209	51	24	205	7	3
Novi Sad	190	86	46	180	11	6
Naples	75	63	84	26	2	8
Geneva	89	30	34	98	3	3
Total	1,832	808	44	1,760	200	11

*Data from James D G, Neville E, Turiaf J, Ballesti J P, et al. A worldwide review of sarcoidosis. Ann NY Acad Sci. 278:321, 1976.

Table 12–3. Results of Calcium Studies in a Series of 818 Patients Related
to Sex, Age of Onset of Sarcoidosis, and Race

	Hypercalcaemia No.	%	Hypercalciuria No.	%
Male	44/203	22	46/76	61
Female	55/344	16	31/116	27
Age of onset (years)				
< 21	2/23	9	2/6	33
21–30	49/224	22	36/80	45
31–40	19/155	12	24/57	42
41–50	17/85	20	10/27	37
>50	12/60	20	5/22	23
English	76/388	20	49/124	40
Irish	7/40	18	7/14	50
West Indian	7/65	11	9/33	27
Other	9/54	17	12/21	57
Total	99/547	18	77/192	40

Note: Normal values—Serum calcium: 9.0–10.5 mg/100 ml (SI 2.20–2.63 mmol/l)
24-hr urine calcium: 100–300 mg (SI 2.5–7.5 mmol/24 hr)

In order to assess how frequently calcium metabolism was abnormal, 75 newly diagnosed sarcoidosis patients had simultaneous serum and urinary calcium levels measured (Table 12–4). Hypercalciuria occurred in 37 patients (49 per cent) and hypercalcaemia in 10 (13 per cent). No patient had a high serum calcium level without a high urinary calcium excretion rate, but hypercalciuria occurred with a normal serum calcium level in 27 (36 per cent) patients. A 24-hour urine collection for measurement of calcium excretion is therefore the most sensitive method of detecting abnormal calicum metabolism.

Our data also suggested that in acute sarcoidosis abnormal calcium metabolism is transient and self-limiting, whereas persistent hypercalciuria, sometimes with hypercalcaemia, is associated with chronic persistent sarcoidosis. Only those with chronic disease had recurrent episodes of renal colic or radiographs showing nephrocalcinosis.

Disordered calcium metabolism is due to overactivity of calcitriol.[2, 3] The natural form, cholecalciferol (vitamin D_3), is metabolised first in the liver to 25-hydroxycholecalciferol, and then a second hydroxy group is added in the kidney to produce the potent, highly active 1,25-dihydroxycholecalciferol (calcitriol). Calcitriol causes increased intestinal calcium absorption, leading to hypercalcaemia and hypercalciuria. This can also be induced by sunlight and can be reversed by steroid therapy.[3] Calcitriol levels correlate with hypercalciuria rather than hypercalcaemia. There is no correlation with parathormone levels[4] (Fig. 12–1).

In a detailed study of 56 sarcoid patients[4], increased parathormone levels were only noted once, a fact that we have also noted in our series. Increased levels of calcitriol despite functional hypoparathyroidism suggest that abnormal calcium metabolism in sarcoidosis is regulated by factors other than parathormone. A sarcoidosis patient with sunshine-induced hypercalcaemia was noted to have raised blood calcitriol levels and also serum immunoreactive parathyroid hormone concentrations in the mid-normal range when they should have been undetectable in the presence of hypercalcaemia. Corticosteroid suppression quickly reduced serum calcium and calcitriol to normal levels and the serum parathyroid levels to low normal. This steroid suppression test is valuable in distinguishing sarcoidosis from sarcoidosis plus primary hyperparathyroidisim.[5] Hypercalcaemia has been reported in

Table 12–4. Simultaneous Determination of Serum and 24-hour Urine Calcium Levels in 75 Patients with Sarcoidosis

Raised Calcium In	No. Patients	%
Serum or urine	37	49
Serum and urine	10	13
Urine only	27	36
Serum only	0	—
Hypercalciuria	37	49
Hypercalcaemia	10	13

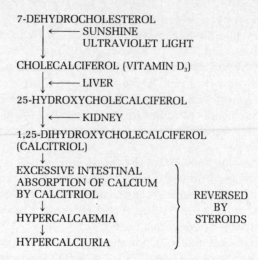

7-DEHYDROCHOLESTEROL
  | ←——— SUNSHINE
  | ULTRAVIOLET LIGHT
  ↓
CHOLECALCIFEROL (VITAMIN D₃)
  | ←——— LIVER
  ↓
25-HYDROXYCHOLECALCIFEROL
  | ←——— KIDNEY
  ↓
1,25-DIHYDROXYCHOLECALCIFEROL
(CALCITRIOL)
  ↓
EXCESSIVE INTESTINAL ⎫
ABSORPTION OF CALCIUM ⎪
BY CALCITRIOL   ⎬ REVERSED
  ↓   ⎪ BY
HYPERCALCAEMIA   ⎪ STEROIDS
  ↓   ⎪
HYPERCALCIURIA   ⎭

Figure 12–1. Abnormal calcium metabolism in sarcoidosis.

an anephric patient with sarcoidosis, with evidence of extrarenal generation of calcitriol in sarcoid tissue itself.

Reiner and colleagues studied calcium metabolism in 13 saroidosis patients with normal renal function, 5 with elevated urinary calcium excretion rates, and none with hypercalcaemia.[7] Calcium hyperabsorption occurred in 6 of those 13 patients when measured by a double isotope method in which 10 μCi of oral calcium[45] and 10 μCi of intravenous calcium[47] were administered simultaneously. The absorption of the oral tracer dose was measured. A clear tendency toward increased bone turnover was shown by calcium kinetic studies in six patients, four of whom were demonstrated to have increased calcium absorption from the gut. These results suggest that in sarcoidosis, abnormalities of calcium metabolism are more common than measurements of serum or urinary calcium alone would suggest.

PHOSPHATE LEVELS

Serum phosphate levels were recorded in 343 patients; they were raised above normal levels in 22 (6 per cent) and were below normal in 25 (7 per cent). No association was demonstrated between abnormal phosphate levels and deranged calcium metabolism.

SERUM PROTEINS AND IMMUNOGLOBULINS

In a worldwide survey of sarcoidosis, serum globulin levels were abnormal in 808 of 1,832 (44 per cent) patients tested[1] (see Table 12–2). In our laboratory serum albumin levels were reduced below 35 gm/1 in 82 of

526 (16 per cent) patients and serum globulin levels were raised above 35 gm/1 in 161 of 526 (31 per cent) patients in the series.

Serum albumin and total protein concentrations were analysed by a Technicon auto-analyser. Qualitative analysis of serum proteins was carried out by zone electrophoresis on cellulose acetate strips.

Abnormal electrophoretic patterns carried no obvious diagnostic or prognostic significance, as no correlation was found with stage of sarcoidosis or the organ system involved.

Immunoglobulin levels were measured in the sera of 71 patients by radial immunodiffusion in buffered agar-gel containing specific antisera. The level of one or more immunoglobulin was raised in 57 of 71 (80 per cent) patients with sarcoidosis; IgG was increased in 43 (56 per cent), IgA in 19 (27 per cent), and IgM in 9 (13 per cent) patients. IgG was increased in one-half of the Caucasian and two-thirds of the West Indian patients. IgA was equally distributed between the two races, but IgM levels were elevated in one-third of the Caucasian and two-thirds of the West Indian patients. There was no significant difference when immunoglobulin levels were compared in acute and chronic sarcoidosis. Abnormal IgG levels bore no special correlation with organ systems involved. There was no significant correlation between immunoglobulin levels and changes in chest radiographs, Kveim-Siltzbach tests, depression of delayed-type hypersensitivity, and hypercalcaemia.

Significant elevations in IgA, IgM, and IgG levels have been noted, with IgM and IgA levels being similarly elevated in Caucasians, Puerto Ricans, and blacks.[8] The IgG levels were highest in black patients and were not elevated among Caucasians. The IgA level was higher in males than in females, but there was no difference in levels between acute and chronic sarcoidosis. When sarcoidosis became inactive, the levels of IgG and IgM fell but the IgA level remained elevated. There was no correlation between immunoglobulin levels and the Kveim-Siltzbach test.

A comparison of immunoglobulin levels in Caucasians and blacks found elevated IgA and IgG levels in blacks with all stages of sarcoidosis, particularly in those with chronic advanced disease, whereas levels were normal in Caucasian subjects.[9] Also observed were significantly high IgA and IgG levels in normal blacks in comparison with healthy Caucasians, whereas IgM were similar. Women of both races tended to have higher IgM levels.

Serum IgD is normally present in very low concentrations in healthy individuals, and up to one-half have undetectable levels. IgD has been detected in the serum of 20 per cent more patients with tuberculosis and in 20 per cent fewer patients with sarcoidosis than in respective controls.[10] High levels of IgD occurred predominantly in older patients with tuberculosis, whereas depression of IgD occurred in middle-aged patients with sarcoidosis. In contrast, another series found normal levels of IgD in patients with sarcoidosis using a radial diffusion technique.[9] In their series, patients with tuberculosis also had markedly elevated levels. Elevated IgD levels have also been noted in leprosy patients and during normal pregnancy.

Bergmann and associates measured IgE levels in 66 patients with sarcoidosis, 20 patients with pulmonary tuberculosis, and 35 normal controls.[11] Although there was considerable overlap, they found significantly higher levels in the sarcoidosis group compared with the tuberculosis and control groups. In contrast, others found that IgE levels were often significantly decreased in patients with sarcoidosis,[12] whereas Tannenbaum and colleagues reported normal IgE levels in their patients.[13]

SERUM ANGIOTENSIN-CONVERTING ENZYME ACTIVITY
(Table 12–5)

Angiotensin-I-converting enzyme (ACE) is a dipeptidyl carboxypeptidase that catalyses the conversion of the decapeptide angiotensin-I to the pressor octapeptide angiotensin-II and the terminal dipeptide I-histidyl-L-leucine. ACE is a membrane-bound glycoprotein located mainly in the pinocytic vesicles of the pulmonary capillary endothelial tissue.[14–16]

Lieberman's original observation in 1974 of raised concentrations of serum angiotensin-converting enzyme (SACE) in 15 out of 17 patients with sarcoidosis focused attention on the enzyme as a biochemical marker for sarcoidosis.[17–19] Worldwide experience from 10 countries was reported at an International Conference on Sarcoidosis in Cardiff,[20] and there have been British reports of the value of SACE activity in various granulomatous disorders.[21–23] Increased activity is thought to reflect stimulation of the monocyte-macrophage system. Circulating blood monocytes, the precursors of epithelioid cells, contain almost no ACE and yet on culture demonstrate the capacity to secrete the enzyme.[24]

Table 12–5. Serum Angiotensin-Converting Enzyme (SACE) Levels in Sarcoidosis and Other Disorders*

Condition	No. Patients	Mean Activity SACE†	Elevated‡ No.	Elevated‡ %
Sarcoidosis (active)	134	98 ± 45	117	87
Sarcoidosis (inactive)	44	38 ± 10	4	9
Primary biliary cirrhosis	31	50 ± 17	9	29
Inflammatory bowel disease	38	31 ± 11	2	5
Lymphoma	35	36 ± 14	4	11
Tuberculosis	59	43 ± 14	14	24
Leprosy	42	38 ± 11	4	9.5
Alcoholic hepatitis	14	32 ± 8	0	—
Lung cancer	55	36 ± 14	7	13
Other respiratory diseases	90	35 ± 10	7	8
Neurological disease	32	39 ± 10	2	6
Diabetes mellitus	24	46 ± 23	3	12.5
Choroidoretinitis	12	31 ± 15	1	8

*Adapted from Dr. P R Studdy's doctoral thesis, submitted to New Castle University.
†nmol/min/ml ± SD.
‡Number and percentage elevated based on those with SACE activity above 52 units.

High turnover granulomas are sites of considerable macrophage activity, and secretory products of this metabolism include not only angiotensin-converting enzyme but also lysozyme, B glucuronidase, and elastase. Immunofluorescent staining has localised ACE and angiotensin-II to epithelioid cells.[24] High concentrations have been noted in sarcoid lymph node tissue.[19, 25] ACE activity has been found in human alveolar macrophages from normal volunteers and patients with pulmonary sarcoidosis. This activity is higher in the alveolar macrophages from smokers than from non-smokers and is even more elevated in sarcoid patients. Compared with alveolar macrophages from normal non-smokers, ACE activity in alveolar macrophages from smokers and patients with sarcoidosis is, respectively, three and five times greater.[26]

SACE has been positively correlated with serum lysozyme levels in sarcoidosis patients.[27, 28] SACE also inactivates bradykinin through hydrolysis of its terminal dipeptide.[29] Increased SACE activity in various diseases involving macrophages in the inflammatory reaction may be related to its inhibitory action on bradykinin, which is a potent inflammatory mediator *in vitro*.[30]

SACE activity is independent of sex, adult age variations, time of day, and eating, but we have noted that it is higher in children age 3 to 15 years. Thus, a higher cutoff point must be taken before a raised value in a child or adolescent can be regarded as significant.

There are several methods of assaying SACE activity, a point worth remembering when comparing results on a global basis. We have found the spectrofluorimetric method of Friedland and Silverstein sensitive and highly reproducible.[31] The dipeptide product L-histidyl-L-leucine formed by the incubation of the test serum and substrate hippuryl-L-histidyl-L-leucine is measured spectrofluorimetrically by the addition of ophthaldialdehyde. Units of activity are expressed as nmol min^{-1} ml^{-1} of dipeptide product formed. Normal serum enzyme activity by this method is 34 ± 9 units (range 16–52 units). Another popular method was described by Lieberman:[18] the unit of activity is described as normoles of hippuric acid released per minute under standard assay conditions.

SACE is produced by endothelial and epithelioid cells predominantly in the pulmonary capillary bed; this localisation has been confirmed by immunoperoxidase and electron microscopy.[32] Purified ACE causes about 50 per cent migration-inhibition of macrophages (but not granulocytes), a phenomenon which is not affected by the specific ACE inhibitor captopril.[33] This seems to be one important role for ACE in sarcoidosis. Captopril does not influence SACE activity in normal subjects nor in those with healed sarcoidosis, but it may magnify the rise in those with active sarcoidosis.[34]

The Fujisoki Pharmaceutical Company of Tokyo has marketed a simple SACE colour test kit that is being evaluated at present. This simple assay is based on colorimetry of the guinoneimine dye produced from the substrate p-hydroxyhippuryl-L-histidyl-L-leucine and an enzyme-induced series of reactions. It is supposedly accurate, extremely simple, and cheap and has good reproducibility.

β2 MICROGLOBULIN

Serum β2 microglobulin is a low–molecular weight protein, associated with histocompatibility antigens and normally found in low levels in serum and other tissue fluids. Raised levels have been reported in patients with sarcoidosis.[35] This, however, is nonspecific, as the protein is also raised in many other diseases.[36, 37] As a marker of cellular activation it could be expected than β2 microglobulin levels would correlate with raised angiotensin-converting enzyme levels,[38] but Parish and colleagues failed to demonstrate any correlation and concluded that the serum β2 microglobulin level is a poor marker of sarcoid disease activity.[39]

LIVER FUNCTION TESTS

Alkaline phosphatase levels were raised in 58 of 252 (23 per cent) patients. We demonstrated no correlation between raised alkaline phosphatase levels or abnormal calcium metabolism and the presence of skeletal changes due to bone cysts in sarcoidosis. However, Reiner and associates investigated 11 patients with sarcoidosis and showed a close correlation between elevated alkaline phosphatase levels and increased radioisotope bone turnover.[7]

We can only speculate that hepatic granulomas were the cause of alkaline phosphatase elevation in some of our patients.

The serum bilirubin level was elevated in 12 (7 per cent) of patients, 164 patients and the serum albumin level reduced in 82 (16 per cent) of 526 patients, but these abnormalities could be accounted for by disorders other than sarcoidosis. For instance, sickle cell disease was a common accompaniment in West Indian sarcoidosis patients.

RENAL FUNCTION TESTS

We obtained no helpful information from routine renal function tests in assessing our sarcoidosis patients. Blood urea levels were transiently elevated in 42 of 213 (20 per cent) patients (see Table 12–1). Chronic renal impairment was only documented in 10 patients in the study population.

URIC ACID LEVELS

Serum uric acid levels were transiently raised in 9 of 50 sarcoidosis patients (see Table 12–1).

This finding may be fortuitous, for no particular association was demonstrated between hyperuricaemia and bone or joint involvement due to sarcoidosis or with other biochemical tests.

Table 12–6. Biochemical Findings in Sarcoidosis

Abnormality	Significance
Hydroxyprolinuria	Indicates acute active disease
Raised serum angiotensin-converting enzyme (SACE) level	Raised in 60% Indicates active epithelioid cell granuloma formation A good monitor of progress and response to steroid therapy
Hyperglobulinaemia	Indicates B cell overactivity by T cell stimulus Particularly elevated in black patients
Raised alkaline phosphatase level	Indicates space-occupying miliary granulomas in liver
Hyperuricaemia	Noted in end-stage renal failure following nephrocalcinosis
Raised serum lysozyme levels	Elevated in sarcoidosis but also nonspecifically in many other conditions including tuberculosis and Crohn's disease Helpful monitor of progress
Hypercalcaemia and hypercalciuria	Transient in the 20- to 30-year age group and persistent in the over-40-year age group

In the differential diagnosis of a patient with punched-out bone cysts, sarcoidosis should be considered if the only suggestion of gout is mild hyperuricaemia.

HYDROXYPROLINURIA

Increased urinary excretion of hydroxyproline has been noted in acute active exudative sarcoidosis but it was normal in the burnt-out fibrotic form of the disease.[40] A fall in the urinary hydroxyproline excretion rate toward normal levels was noted with time in all subjects studied serially, irrespective of treatment, and this fall was also associated with a fall of serum alkaline phosphatase levels.

The significance of abnormal biochemical findings in sarcoidosis is summarised in Table 12–6.[41]

REFERENCES

1. James DG, Neville E, Turiaf J, Battesti JP, et al. A worldwide review of sarcoidosis. Ann NY Acad Sci. 278:321, 1976.
2. Bell NH, Stern PH, Pantzer E, Sinhat K, Deluca HF. Evidence that increased circulating 1.25 dihydroxyvitamin D is the probable cause for abnormal calcium metabolism in sarcoidosis. J Clin Invest. 64:218, 1979.
3. Zerwekh J, Pak CYC, Kaplan RA, McGuire JL, Upchurch K, Breslau N, Johnson R. Pathogenic role of 1.25-dihydroxyvitamin D in sarcoidosis and absorptive hypercalciuria. Different response to prednisolone therapy. J Clin Endocrinol Metab. 51:381, 1980.
4. Handslip PD, Bone M, Woodhead JS, Davies BH. Calcium and phosphate metabolism in sarcoidosis with particular reference to parathyroid function. Br J Dis Chest. 75:55, 1980.

5. Ghose RR, Woodhead JS, Brown, RC. Incomplete suppression of parathyroid hormone activity in sarcoidosis presenting with hypercalcaemia. Postgrad Med J. 59:572, 1983.
6. Barbour GL, Coburn JW, Slatopolsky E, Norman AW, Horst RL. Hypercalcaemia in an anephric patient with sarcoidosis. Evidence for extrarenal generation of 1.25 dihydroxyvitamin D. N Engl J Med. 305:440, 1981.
7. Reiner M, Sigurdsson G, Nunziata V, Malik MA, Poole GW, Jepiin GF. Abnormal calcium metabolism in normocalcaemic sarcoidosis. Br Med J. 2:1473, 1976.
8. Celikoglu S, Vieira LO, Siltzbach LE. Serum immunoglobulin levels in sarcoidosis. In Levinsky L, Macholda F (ed): Vth Internat Conf Sarcoidosis. Praha, Universita Karlova. p 168, 1971.
9. Goldstein RA, Israel HL, Rawnsley RM. Effect of race and stage of disease on the serum immunoglobulilns in sarcoidosis. In Levinsky L, Macholda F (eds): Vth Internat Conf Sarcoidosis. Praha, Universita Karlova. p 178, 1971.
10. Buckley CE, Trayer HR. Serum IgD concentrations in sarcoidosis and tuberculosis. Clin Exp Immunol. 10:257, 1972.
11. Bergmann von KCh, Zaumseil I, Lachmann B. IgE konzentrationen im serum von patienten mit sarkoidose und lungen tuberkulose. Dtsch Gesundheit Wes. 27:1774, 1972.
12. Yagura T, Shimizu M, Yamamura Y, Tachibana T. Serum IgE levels and reaginic type skin reactions in sarcoidosis. Clin Exp Immunol. 21:289, 1975.
13. Tannenbaum H, Rocklin RE, Schur PH, Scheffer AL. Immunological identification of subpopulations of mononuclear cells in sarcoid granulomas. Ann NY Acad Sci. 278:236, 1976.
14. Hodge RL, Ng KKF, Vane JR. Disappearance of angiotensin from the circulation of the dog. Nature 215:138, 1967.
15. Ng KKF, Vane JR. Fate of angiotensin I in the circulation. Nature 218:144, 1968.
16. Ryan US, Ryan JW, Whitaker C, Chiu A. Localisation of angiotensin converting enzyme (kinase II) imunocytochemistry and immunofluorescence. Tissue Cell. 8:125, 1976.
17. Lieberman J. A new confirmatory test for sarcoidosis. Am Rev Resp Dis. 109:743, 1974.
18. Lieberman J. Elevation of serum angiotensin-converting-enzyme (ACE) levels in sarcoidosis. Am J Med 59:365, 1975.
19. Lieberman J. The specificity and nature of serum angiotensin converting enzyme (serum ACE) elevations in sarcoidosis. Ann NY Acad Sci 278:488, 1976.
20. Studdy P, James DG, et al. Serum angiotensin converting enzyme (SACE) experience in ten centers. In Jones Williams W, Davies BH (eds): Sarcoidosis. Cardiff, Alpha and Omega Press. p 241, 1980.
21. Ashutosh K, Keighley JFH. Diagnostic value of serum angiotensin converting enzyme activity in lung disease. Thorax. 31:552, 1976.
22. Studdy P, Bird R, James DG, Sherlock S. Serum angiotensin converting enzyme (SACE) in sarcoidosis and other granulomatous disorders. Lancet 2:1331, 1978.
23. Khuory F, Teasdale PR, Smith D, Jones OG, Carter JR. Angiotensin converting enzyme in sarcoidosis: A British study. Br J Dis Chest. 73:382, 1979.
24. Silverstein E, Friedland J, Pertshuk LP. Sarcoidosis pathogenesis. Mechanism of angiotensin converting enzyme elevation: Epithelioid cell localisation and induction in macrophages and monocytes in culture. In Jones Williams W, Davies BH (eds): Sarcoidosis. Cardiff, Alpha and Omega Press. p 246, 1980.
25. Silverstein E, Friedland J, Lyons HA, Gourin A. Markedly elevated converting enzyme in lymph nodes containing non necrotizing granulomas in sarcoidosis. Proc Natl Acad Sci (USA). 73:2137, 1976.
26. Hinman LE, Stevens CA, JBL. Angiotensin convertase activities in human alveolar macrophages, effects of cigarette smoking and sarcoidosis. Science 205:202, 1979.
27. Silverstein E, Friedland J, Lyons HA, Gourin A. Elevation of angiotensin converting enzyme in granulomatous lymph nodes and serum in sarcoidosis, clinical and possible pathogenic significance. Ann NY Acad Sci. 278:498, 1976.
28. Selroos O, Tiitien H, Gronhagen-Riska F, Fyhrquist F, Klockars M. Angiotensin converting enzyme and lysozyme in sarcoidosis. In Jones Williams W, Davies BH (eds): Sarcoidosis. Cardiff, Alpha and Omega Press. p 303, 1980.
29. Erods EG. Angiotensin I converting enzyme. Cir Res. 36:247, 1975.
30. Gronhagen-Riska G. Angiotensin converting enzyme. Scand J Resp Dis. 60:83, 1979.
31. Friedland J, Silverstein E. A sensitive fluorimetric assay for serum angiotensin converting enzyme. Am J Clin Pathol. 66:416, 1976.

32. Silverstein E, Friedland J, Stanck AE, Smith PR, Deason Dr, Lyon HA. Pathogenesis of sarcoidosis. Mechanism of angiotensin converting enzyme elevation. T lymphocyte modulation of enzyme induction in mononuclear phagocytes enzyme properties. *In* Chretien J, Marsac J, Saltiel JC (eds): Proc 9th Internat Conf Sarcoidosis. Paris, Pergamon Press. p 319, 1983.
33. Gronhagen-Riska C, Fyrquist F, Pettersson T, Welin MG, Weber TH. Leucocyte migration inhibitory effect of purified human lung angiotensin converting enzyme. *In* Chretien J, Marsac J, Saltiel JC (eds): Proc 9th Internat Conf Sarcoidosis. Paris, Pergamon Press. p 326, 1983.
34. Ueda T, Tachibana T, Kokuba T, Yamamoto Y, Yoshida N. Further evaluation of serum angiotensin converting enzyme activity in active sarcoidosis with captopril administration. *In* Chretien J, Marsac J, Saltiel JC (eds): Proc 9th Internat Conf Sarcoidosis. Paris, Pergamon Press. p 475, 1983.
35. Mornex JE, Revillard JP, Vincento Detie XP, Brune J. Elevated serum microglobulin levels and CLq binding immune complexes in sarcoidosis. Biomedicine. 31:210, 1979.
36. Teasdale C, Mander AM, Fifield R, Keyser JW, Newcombe RG, Hughes LE. Serum $\beta2$ microglobulin in controls and cancer patients. Clin Chem Acta. 78:135, 1977.
37. Talal N, Grey HM, Zyaifler N, Michaiski J, Danieis T. Elevated salivary and synovial fluid $\beta2$ microglobulin in Sjogren's syndrome and rheumatoid arthritis. Science. 187:1196, 1975.
38. Mornex JF, Biot N, Pacheco Y, Perrin Fayolle M, Vincent C, Revilland JP. $\beta2$ microglobulin levels in serum and bronchoalveolae lavage fluid from patients with sarcoidosis. *In* Chretien J, Marsac J, Saltiel JC (eds): Proc 9th Internat Conf Sarcoidosis. Paris, Pergamon Press. p 372, 1983.
39. Parish RW, Williams JD, Davies BH. Serum $\beta2$ microglobulin and angiotensin converting enzyme activity in sarcoidosis. Thorax. 37:936, 1982.
40. Massaro D, Handler AE, Katz S, Young RC. Excretion of hydroxyproline in patients with sarcoidosis. Am Rev Resp Dis. 93:929, 1966.
41. Studdy PR, Bird R, Neville E, James DG. Biochemical findings in sarcoidosis. J Clin Pathol. 33:528, 1980.

13

Immunology

Sarcoidosis is characterised by dysfunction of circulating T cells and overactivity of B cells.[1] Activated macrophages and T helper cells are conjointly responsible for activation of B lymphocytes and immunoglobulin synthesis at sites of activity, such as the lungs in sarcoidosis (or the synovium in rheumatoid arthritis or the skin in mycosis fungoides). Associated features are the presence of circulating immune complexes, various changes in serum complement levels, enhanced K and NK cell activity, and certain HLA correlations. There is increased recognition of cell types in blood and broncho-alveolar fluid and also of enzymes and proteins associated with these cell types. Some are proving to be helpful markers of activity (see Chapter 14).

ANERGY

Patients with sarcoidosis fail to respond to tuberculin and other antigens, including dinitrochlorobenzene.[2] They show depression of delayed-type hypersensitivity due to hyper-reactivity of circulating T lymphocytes, particularly T suppressor cells. Cutaneous anergy is closely mirrored by *in vitro* cellular hyporeactivity to phytohaemagglutinin. It has been postulated that sarcoid lymphocytes are inherently normal and that the impaired response is due to inhibitory factors in the patient's serum.[3] Circulating immune complexes affect T lymphocytes and may contribute to this anergy characterised by a low OKT4:OKT8 ratio.

CELLULAR IMMUNITY

Monoclonal antibody techniques have enabled the proportions of helper (Tm) to suppressor (Tg) T cells in peripheral blood and broncho-alveolar lavage fluid to be compared in patients with active and inactive sarcoidosis and also in patients with idiopathic pulmonary fibrosis and in normal control subjects. Pulmonary sarcoidosis is a disorder mediated by excess helper T lymphocyte activity at sites of disease activity.[4, 5] The most striking difference is that the T helper:suppressor ratio is 10.5:1 in active pulmonary sarcoidosis

174

compared with 1.4:1 in inactive disease. There are twice as many helper cells in the lungs as in the blood, whereas suppressor cells remain conspicuous in the peripheral blood. It seems as though the activated helper cells have been mobilised to the sites of disease activity, such as the lungs, leaving behind anergic suppressor cells in the peripheral blood (Table 13–1).

Clinicians in the Italian school are extending these observations to the redistribution of T cells throughout the body, in keeping with the multisystem nature of the disease.[6-8] The excess helper T cells are evident in the lungs, lymph nodes, skin, eyes (conjunctival nodules and aqueous humour), and liver. Also intriguing is their demonstration of a defined immunological pattern (T helper phenotype) in lung parenchyma at an early phase when transbronchial lung biopsies are still free of granulomas. These studies support earlier suggestions that alveolitis precedes granuloma formation and also suggest that the excess T helper cells are disseminated early enough in various tissues to stimulate B cell activity to produce immunoglobulins.

T lymphocytes seem to modulate the induction of angiotensin-converting enzyme (ACE) in monocytes in culture and may play a role in inducing ACE synthesis in epithelioid cells in sarcoidosis.[9] There is a good correlation between increased SACE activity and the increased level of broncho-alveolar lymphocytes (BAL) in sarcoidosis, whereas extrinsic allergic alveolitis is characterised by an increased BAL with normal SACE.[10] In sarcoidosis, T cells in the lungs provide mediator release for monocyte chemotactic factor and migration inhibitor factors and also help B cell immunoglobulin production.

Beta$_2$ microglobulin ($\beta_2 m$) is a low–molecular weight protein (11,800 daltons) that constitutes part of the HLA antigens on cell membranes. It is released at a constant rate in normal subjects, but activated T cells release $\beta_2 m$ from both T and B cells. Raised levels have been detected in both serum and broncho-alveolar fluid in sarcoid patients compared with controls but with no agreed relationship to radiological stage or clinical activity.[11-13] It does not correlate closely with SACE activity, suggesting a disparity between

Table 13–1. The OKT4:OKT8 Ratio in Sarcoidosis and Other Disorders

OKT4 (Helper) High (> 2 : 1)	OKT8 Ratio (Suppressor) Low (< 1:1)
Leprosy : Tuberculoid	Lepromatous
Sarcoid : Skin	Blood
Kveim	Negative tuberculin
Lung	
Rheumatoid : synovium	Lymph node
Graft v. host : acute	Chronic
Chronic active hepatitis : HBsAg negative	HBsAg positive
Behçet's disease—active; inactive	Preactive
Guillain-Barré syndrome	Rhinoscleroma
Asbestosis	Homosexuality
	AIDS
	Suntan

granulomatous macrophage (SACE) activity and lymphocyte (β_2m) activation.[11]

Ia antigens, usually present on lymphoid cells of non-T origin, are also expressed in a small proportion of circulating T cells. They may be identified by indirect immunofluorescence using a monoclonal antibody to framework determinants of HLA-Ia–like antigens. Ia-T cells are significantly increased in the circulation in sarcoidosis, and this increase is much more evident in the active compared with the inactive stage of the disease.[14]

ACTIVATED MACROPHAGES

Macrophages, derived from bone marrow monocytes, are mononuclear phagocytes with abundant cytoplasm and numerous processes. The cytoplasm shows variable organelles, increasing in number and complexity with the degree of cell activity. Microtubules, Golgi complexes, and various membrane-bound vesicles, lysosomes, and residual bodies are frequent. Mitochondria are numerous, and both smooth and rough endoplasmic reticulum are present. The cell membrane is characteristically thrown into folds and processes, which, together with pinocytic and phagocytic vesicles, indicates their essentially mobile phagocytic nature.

Following an antigenic stimulus, monocytes residing in the lung interstitium become activated alveolar macrophages. There are many known stimulators of pulmonary macrophage activity, such as exogenous mycobacteria, parasites, silica, beryllium, and endogenous lipopolysaccharides and haemosiderin.[15] The stimulus that leads to multisystem sarcoidosis remains an enigma. The mediator release provided by these macrophages contributes lymphocyte-activating factor and fibroblast growth factor.[16] Mononuclear cells from the circulating blood of sarcoidosis patients emit high levels of chemoluminescence upon ingestion of zymosan. The response of sarcoid cells is higher than that observed in cells of normal controls or from those of recovered sarcoidosis patients or patients with tuberculosis.[17]

Macrophages (and probably epithelioid cells) play a crucial role in T lymphocyte differentiation and activation in the process of cellular immunity. They play a role in both the afferent limb of the immune responses and as effector cells by phagocytosis, with presentation of antigens to lymphocytes and with the production of many soluble products. Monocytes secrete prostaglandins, which, in turn, activate glass-adherent T suppressor cells to release a peptide that suppresses T and B cell mitogen response.[18]

EPITHELIOID CELLS

Activated macrophages clump together densely into giant and epithelioid cells. These epithelioid cells are mononuclear cells with pale vacuolated cytoplasm and complex interdigitating cell processes. On light microscopy and histochemistry they are morphologically indistinguishable in sarcoidosis,

Kveim granulomas, tuberculosis, chronic beryllium disease, and extrinsic allergic alveolitis. Electron microscopy confirms this similarity and shows that the most prominent features are numerous membrane-bound muco-glycoprotein-containing vesicles and associated Golgi complexes.[19] Epithelioid cells may be phagocytic or secretory, depending on the activating stimulus and defense mechanisms in the host. They secrete angiotensin-converting enzyme (ACE), calcitriol, lysozyme, collagenase, and several other enzymes important to the success of an inflammatory reaction. The epithelioid cell localisation of ACE has been confirmed by immunoperoxidase and electron microscopy.[9]

Histochemistry may permit differentiation of acute from chronic sarcoidosis. Cryostat sections of sarcoid lymph nodes have been examined and enzyme activity assessed by estimating acid phosphatase and leucine-aminopeptidase. High activity of both enzymes is associated with rapid resolution of the sarcoid process and a good prognosis, whereas low enzyme activity reflects chronicity of the disease.[20]

K AND NK CELL ACTIVITY

Killer (K) cells are non-immune effector cells that may destroy antibody-coated target cells; this is recognised as antibody-dependent cell-mediated cytotoxicity. Natural killer (NK) cells are similar but destroy target cells without antibody; this is known as spontaneous lymphocyte-mediated cytotoxicity. Both K and NK cell activities are higher in sarcoidosis than in controls and in active compared with inactive disease. Activity is more pronounced with advanced pulmonary involvement. There is a good correlation between K cell activity and elevated SACE and lysozyme activity.[21]

These changes may, however, be epiphenomena of chronic inflammation. It has been shown experimentally that products of activated macrophages, possibly interferon, play an essential role in NK cell activation.[22] Similar increased NK cell activity has also been demonstrated in patients with active tuberculosis as compared with normal control subjects.[23]

HUMORAL IMMUNITY

B Cells

Whereas there may be both impairment and enhancement of cellular immunity, there is always enhanced humoral immunity with raised immunoglobulin levels; increased circulating antibody titres to Epstein-Barr virus, herpes simplex, rubella, measles, and parainfluenza viruses, and to chlamydia; increased antibody responses to mismatched blood; and occasional false-positive Wassermann reactions. Associated with raised immunoglobulin levels are elevations of kappa and lambda free light chains. In a series of 63 patients with sarcoidosis, light chains were measured by radioimmunoassay and found to be elevated in 79 per cent with chronic active disease over two years duration compared with 10 per cent of those with recent active disease and only 1 per cent of those with healed inactive disease. Elevated light chains indicate B cell overactivity and are markers of chronicity in sarcoidosis.[24] Broncho-alveolar fluid shows an increase of IgG, IgM, and IgA as a result of B cell overactivity in sarcoidosis.

Complement

The levels of total serum complement and of C_3, C_4, and C_5 degradation products have been highly variable in different series, partly because of the variability in clinical material and the differences between acute and chronic sarcoidosis. Analysis of the literature and a personal series[25] indicates that significant falls in C_3 and C_4 levels were particularly evident in those with hyperglobulinaemia. Very low levels of C_3 were noted in 8 of 30 patients.

Broncho-Alveolar Fluid (BAL)

In addition to the increase of activated macrophages, there is also an increase of protein markers of inflammation in sarcoidosis. BAL shows a sharp increase of α 1-antitrypsin and a smaller increase of orosomucoid compared with controls, whereas haptoglobulin and C-reactive protein levels have been noted to rise more obviously in serum. There seems to be a dissociation between these inflammatory protein responses in the alveoli and in serum.[26] The dissociation is even greater when the enzymes elastase, lactic dehydrogenase, glucuronidase, lysozyme, acid phosphatase, and amylase are compared in BAL and serum. The enzyme BAL:serum ratio is higher than the protein ratio. It is likely that some protein production may be local.[27] Yet another protein, provisionally termed L1, may provide another measure of activity of sarcoidosis. It is produced by stimulated macrophages and is measured by sensitive radioimmunoassay.[28] Just as ACE is elevated in serum (SACE) in active sarcoidosis, so is it elevated in broncho-alveolar fluid (LACE). There is a good correlation between SACE and LACE when sarcoidosis is essentially intrathoracic. With disseminated extrathoracic involvement there is an even greater rise in LACE and its correlation with SACE disappears.[29] Increased levels of neutrophils and histamine in BAL have been noted in patients with pulmonary fibrotic sarcoidosis, so further studies are needed to determine whether these factors are fibrogenic or reflect an unfavourable course toward fibrosis.[30]

Circulating Immune Complexes (CIC)

Various techniques have been employed to detect circulating immune complexes (CIC). They are most evident at the stage of erythema nodosum, iritis, polyarthralgia, and bilateral hilar lymphadenopathy in which C_3 activation products have been found within the first six weeks. During this early stage of acute sarcoidosis there is activation of the complement system due to circulating immune complexes. These tests for circulating complexes subside as the acute skin lesions disappear. Whenever they are detectable, the sedimentation rate is very high, so this remains the cheapest bedside indicator of these complexes.

Using a variety of methods, CIC will be detected in about one-half of all patients with sarcoidosis. As one might expect, higher levels are found in active disease,[31-33] and close correlations have also been made with chest x-ray Stage 2 or 3[34, 35] or to neither.[36] These differences may be related to variations in the composition of CIC; acute disease is related to IgG-predominant complexes and chronicity with complement-fixing IgG complexes.[37] There is no obvious correlation between CIC and SACE, but the presence of CIC correlates significantly with low levels of circulating T-suppressor lymphocytes. In limited studies it has been claimed that immune complexes are present within granulomas[38] and shown by others to be confined to the pulmonary interstitium.[39] It is uncertain whether these findings are specific or incidental. The relationship of high immunoglobulin levels to the formation of immune complexes and granulomas has recently been highlighted by studies of experimental BCG granulomas. Antibody excess, in particular IgM, combined with BCG appears to be bacteriostatic with the production of small, non-necrotic, rapidly healing granulomas. In contrast, antibody combined with BCG at equivalence causes early necrotic lesions with abscesses rather than granulomas.[40]

Immune Response Serum Suppressor Factors

There is increasing recognition of many serum suppressor factors.[3, 41-47] They are present in sarcoid sera but also in normal and other disease states. Both low– and high–molecular weight suppressor factors have recently been demonstrated; the latter is probably an immune complex. It activates normal T suppressor cells, and its levels are inversely correlated with T suppressor cell numbers.[48]

Kveim-Siltzbach Skin Test

Historically the test has been widely used and is of proven value in diagnosis (see Chapter 1 and Table 3–2).[49]

Kveim-Siltzbach "antigen" is a saline suspension of human sarcoid tissue prepared from the spleen of a patient suffering from active sarcoidosis. The antigen, 0.15 ml, is injected intradermally very superficially into the flexor surface of the forearm, and the inoculation site is observed for the development of a visible and palpable nodule during the ensuing four to six weeks. Any palpable nodule is biopsied, usually one month after the injection, using a Hayes-Martin drill. This core of tissue is serially sectioned for evidence of sarcoid tissue or a foreign body–giant cell reaction; this decision is made blind, that is, without knowledge of the clinical picture. A Kveim-Siltzbach test is reported as positive if the intradermally injected antigen produces a nodule in the course of three to six weeks, and this nodule shows evidence of sarcoid tissue as distinct from a foreign body–giant cell reaction (Fig. 13–1; see also color plate 7). This skin test is positive in about three-fourths of patients with active disease and is therefore a useful diagnostic marker.

Attempts have also been made to develop *in vitro* Kveim tests.[50, 51] These tests measure the transformation or macrophage/leucocyte migration inhibition factors of lymphocytes cultured with Kveim preparations. The *in vitro* tests have the advantages of a rapid result, within two to three days, and the avoidance of biopsies and problems in histological diagnosis. The results, however, have been inconsistent[52–54] and have led to doubt regarding the "antigenicity" of the Kveim preparation and even the role of delayed hypersensitivity in the reaction. These tests have thus far not lived up to their early promise and have largely been discontinued.

The active Kveim principle remains unknown. It has been claimed that the active fraction is present in dense lysosomes[55]; it is very stable, resisting a variety of extraction processes including defatting and peptic digestion.[56] It is presumed to be antigenic, and the reaction is that of hypersensitivity. A parallel may be drawn between the Kveim test and the beryllium patch test in beryllium disease, the zirconium skin reaction in patients with zirconium deodorant granulomas, and the lepromin reaction in leprosy. All are individually specific for their own disease state (Table 13–2). They are all

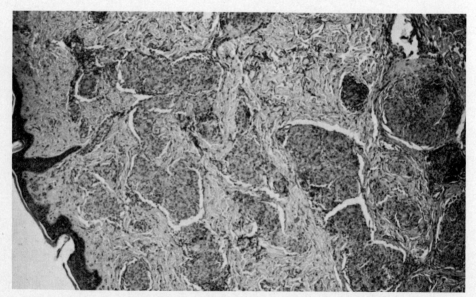

Figure 13–1. Positive Kveim-Siltzbach skin test showing sarcoid granulomas. H & E × 200.

Table 13–2. Skin Tests in Which a Sarcoid Granuloma Develops One Month After Inoculation

Skin Test	Antigen	How Done	Read At	Positive Result	Negative Result	Interpretation of Results and Remarks
Kveim-Siltzbach	Human sarcoid tissue from spleen or lymph node	Intradermal	1 month	Palpable nodule biopsy reveals sarcoid tissue	Suggests either sarcoidosis not present or inactive	Positive test in 80% of patients with sarcoidosis. Also indicates activity
Zirconium	1:10,000 solution zirconium chloride or nitrate	Intradermal	1 month	Palpable nodule biopsy reveals sarcoid tissue	Rules out zirconium hypersensitivity	Specific for zirconium hypersensitivity
Beryllium	1% beryllium sulphate or nitrate	Patch	2 days and 1 month	Eczematous rash; Palpable nodule biopsy reveals sarcoid tissue	Rules out beryllium hypersensitivity	Specific for beryllium hypersensitivity
Lepromin					Negative in lepromatous leprosy	Aid to classification and prognosis rather than diagnosis of leprosy
—Fernandez	Skin bacilli	Intradermal	2 days	Tuberculin-like		
—Mitsuda	Extract of nodules of lepromatous leprosy	Intradermal	1 month	Biopsy of palpable nodule reveals sarcoid tissue		

forms of hypersensitivity, as they occur only in patients who have been in contact with the causative agent. The tests are negative prior to exposure, a positive result is obtained with very high dilutions, and the reaction is specific.

Several factors influence the Kveim-Siltzbach reaction, which must still be regarded as a crude but most useful biological test. Potent antigen is essential, and this means that it must be obtained from the spleen of a patient with active sarcoidosis. Another important factor is the histologist's interpretation of the biopsy material, for an inexperienced observer could confuse sarcoid tissue with a nonspecific foreign body–giant cell reaction, particularly if doubly refractile crystals are not sought by polarised light. Finally, the Kveim-Siltzbach test reaction is suppressed by oral corticosteroids, just as any sarcoid tissue is suppressed by these potent anti-inflammatory agents. An occasional false-positive result is inevitable with a biological test of this kind, but a figure of less than 2 per cent is acceptable.

It is particularly helpful when histological confirmation is otherwise lacking or equivocal. It is useful in the differential diagnosis of diffuse pulmonary mottling, uveitis, or erythema nodosum, and it is also worth performing in obscure cases of subacute meningitis or cranial nerve palsies. It is negative in patients with non-specific local sarcoid tissue reactions and all other granulomatous disorders.

The Kveim-Siltzbach test is well recognised as a diagnostic marker of sarcoidosis and is of value in assessing activity of the disease. Antigens from different centres produce a similar high rate of positive reactions in active (radiographical Stages I and II) disease, varying from 75[57] to 86 per cent.[58] In chronic (radiographical Stage III) disease with a duration of more than two years, the positive rate is lower, ranging from 34[58] to 55 per cent.[57]

HLA Antigens

We have studied the distribution of inherited histocompatibility (HLA) antigens in sarcoidosis patients with erythema nodosum, polyarthritis, uveitis, lupus pernio, and bone cysts. The HLA antigens were identified within 24 hours of venipuncture using a modified two-stage lymphotoxicity micro method, testing the lymphocytes of patients for 22 different antigens.[59] In a series of 107 patients with histologically proven sarcoidosis, there was no overall perturbation of frequency of HLA antigens (Table 13–3). However, B8 was significantly associated with sarcoid arthritis and erythema nodosum whether alone or in combination. Because of the linkage disequilibrium between A1 and B8, A1 increased in association with arthritis. Of 52 patients with acute sarcoidosis, B8 was present in 26 (50 per cent; $p = 0.02$), but when those with either arthritis or erythema nodosum are removed only 5 of 21 (24 per cent) remain; that is, B8 is not associated with acute sarcoidosis itself. Similarly, when the same patients are excluded from the group who

Table 13–3. HLA Types and Their Significance in Sarcoidosis*

HLA Type	Significance in Sarcoidosis
B8/A1	Sarcoid arthritis erythema nodosum
B13	Chronicity
CW7	Sarcoidosis in English
B8/CW7/DR3	Good prognosis in sarcoidosis in English (but not West Indians)
DR3	Short duration of disease
B7	Symptomatic tuberculin-negative Swedish
BW15	Black Americans

*Data from Neville E, James, DG, Brewerton DA, James DCO, Cockburn C, Fenichal B. HLA antigens and features of sarcoidosis. *In* Jones Williams W, Davies BH (eds): Sarcoidosis. Cardiff, Alpha and Omega Press. p 201, 1980.

achieved chest x-ray resolution, B8 is only found in 4 patients of 22 (18 per cent).

Of 55 patients with chronic sarcoidosis, six (11 per cent) were HLA-B13 (p = 0.002); this was also significant when chronic was compared with acute sarcoidosis (p = 0.034). B17 also occurred in six patients (11 per cent) from the chronic sarcoid population, but this did not achieve statistical significance.

In this same group of patients, further studies were made of HLA A, B, C, and DR typing, comparing findings in English and West Indian patients and also comparing patients with acute and chronic sarcoidosis.[60] English patients who are B8/CW7/DR3 have a significantly increased frequency, and West Indians who are DR7 are at relative risk. The B8/CW7/DR3 haplotype is significantly associated with good prognosis and short duration of disease in English patients. There was no association between any HLA antigen and prognosis in West Indian patients (see Table 13–3).

Other studies indicate a normal overall distribution of HLA antigens in familial sarcoidosis,[61] but clinical features were sometimes not selected. In Sweden HLA-B7 predominated in Caucasians, who were more likely to be tuberculin-negative and symptomatic. In black patients in South Carolina there was also a suggestion of an overall increase in HLA-B7 but this was not confirmed in Washington, where, instead, it was noted that sarcoidosis occurred 5.5 times more frequently among BW15 individuals when compared with those lacking that antigen.[62] However, the presence of HLA-BW15 did not correlate with specific disease manifestation. In a large series of 100 black patients from Baltimore,[63] the disease was associated with HLA-AW30. The close link demonstrated between HLA-B8 and erythema nodosum may explain in part the different frequencies with which erythema nodosum is observed in sarcoidosis populations around the world. In the three British series, erythema nodosum was reported in 31 per cent, whereas B8 was found in 29 per cent of the population. In Japan, erythema nodosum was unusual (4 per cent), and B8 was present in less than 2 per cent of the general population. Despite this good correlation in the series at either end of the scale, it is not as convincing when extended to other series. British

Caucasians who have HLA-B8 and who develop sarcoidosis are likely to express it with arthritis or erythema nodosum or both. Not all patients with these manifestations of sarcoidosis have B8, and not all with B8 will develop these lesions; clearly other factors are also operative (Fig. 13–2).

AUTO-IMMUNITY

There are certain well-recognised indicators of an auto-immune disorder. Sarcoidosis does not fulfill all these criteria satisfactorily. There is one pattern of sarcoidosis that could conceivably fit, namely, erythema nodosum with hilar adenopathy, a syndrome that may be associated with a circulating immune complex. Auto-antibodies are infrequent in sarcoidosis compared with other disorders (Table 13–4).

PATHOGENESIS

The sarcoid granuloma is a battleground between antigen and the cellular and humoral defenses of the body. Macrophages are stimulated by the antigenic attack and eventually coalesce into giant cells and epithelioid cell granulomas (Fig. 13–3). T helper cells are mobilised to this point of activity and co-operate with macrophages, leading to B cell overactivity. The T cells

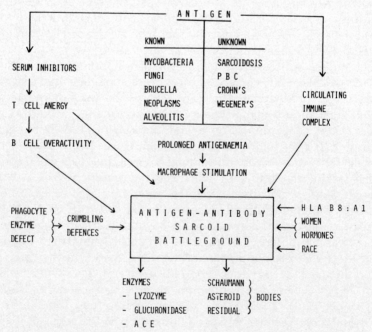

Figure 13–2. Factors contributing to sarcoid granuloma formation.

Table 13–4. Auto-antibodies in Patients with Liver Granulomas

Patients	Antimitochondrial Antibody			Smooth Muscle Antibody			Antinuclear Antibody		
		Positive			*Positive*			*Positive*	
	Tested	*No.*	*%*	*Tested*	*No.*	*%*	*Tested*	*No.*	*%*
Primary biliary cirrhosis	24	19	79	13	6	22	18	5	27
Sarcoidosis	23	1	4	2	0	0	6	0	0
Miscellaneous	3	0	0	5	2	40	8	1	12
Undiagnosed	5	0	0	4	2	50	6	2	33
Overall	55	20	36	24	10	41	38	8	21

provide various lymphokines, and the B cells produce immunoglobulins and various antibodies. The enzymes secreted by the granuloma include angiotensin-converting enzyme, lysozyme, glucuronidase, collagenase, and elastase. With aging, the granulomas are infiltrated by fibroblasts, and early fibrosis is recognised by increasing deposition of reticulin, which is gradually replaced by collagen, which in turn is transformed into structureless eosinophilic hyaline material.

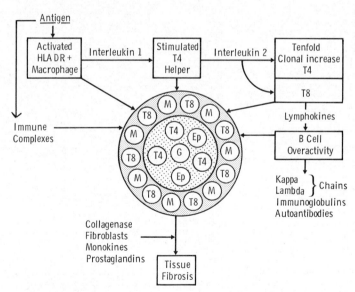

Figure 13–3. Sarcoid granuloma formation.

Activated macrophages within various sarcoid granulomas are now being fingerprinted by a combination of immunofluorescent and histochemical techniques and by monoclonal antibodies directed against antigen-presenting macrophage subsets. This dynamic approach should lead to a better understanding of the basic molecular biology and also toward the aetiology of sarcoidosis.[64, 65]

Macrophages with the phenotype HLA-DR +, RFD-2 +, acid phosphatase (ACP) +/−, adenosine triphosphatase (ATPase) +/− make up 66 per cent of the cell population of the sarcoid granuloma; the remainder are T cells. The suppressor-cytotoxic T8 cells are limited to the periphery of the granuloma, whereas the T4 cells are found throughout the granuloma. The T4:T8 ratio is on the order of 5:1 to 3:1. The same configuration is observed in the Kveim granuloma. We are now able to recognise three different types of macrophages in the sarcoid granuloma (Table 13–5).

Table 13–5. Frequency and Distribution of Cell Types in Sarcoid and Kveim Granulomas*

Cell Type	Phenotype†	Sarcoid/Kveim Granuloma‡
T	UCHT1 + HLA-DR − TO 15 −	40%
OKT4:T8 Ratio	OKT4:OKT8	5:1
Macrophages	HLA-DR + RFD-2 + RFD-1 − ACP + ATPase ±	66%
Activated macrophages and epithelioid and giant cells	As above	50%
Interdigitating cells	HLA-DR + RFD-2 − ACP − ATPase + RFD-1 +	50%
Tissue histiocytes	HLA-DR − RFD-2 + ACP − ATPase ± RFD-1 −	Occasional

*Data from Mishra BB, Poulter LW, Janossy, G, James DG. The distribution of lymphoid- and macrophage-like cell subsets of sarcoid and Kveim granulomata; possible mechanism of negative PPD reaction in sarcoidosis. Clin Exp Immunol. 54:705, 1983.
†Key: UCHT—University College Hospital.
        TO 15—B cell monoclonal antibody.
        RFD—Royal Free Hospital.
        ACP—Acid phosphatase.
        ATPase—Adenosine triphosphatase.
‡Percentages represent proportion of total lymphoid cells or of total non-lymphoid cells in granuloma.

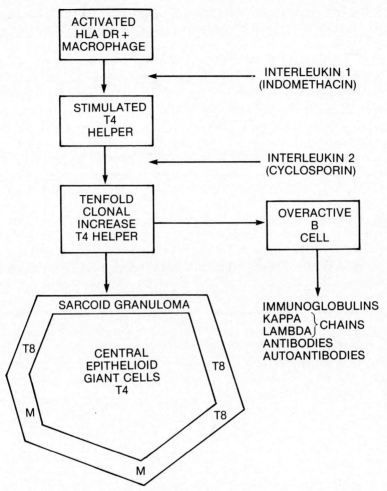

Figure 13–4. Influence of interleukins on granuloma formation.

The periphery contains a large number of antigen-presenting interdigi-tating (ID) cells similar to those found in the lymph node paracortex and at the cortico-medullary junction of the thymus. The centre of the granuloma consists of epithelioid and giant cells, which are derived from macrophages. Tissue histiocytes, the third type, are occasionally seen, are more diffusely distributed in the granuloma, and are not even restricted to the granuloma itself. There is evidence of synergism between the interdigitating cells and T8 cells in the periphery of the granuloma and the epithelioid cells with T4 cells in their centre.[64] This pattern is also seen in skin biopsies of patients with tuberculoid leprosy but not in those with lepromatous leprosy. It is suggested that the architectural aggregation of T lymphocyte subpopulations in the tuberculoid leprosy granuloma is immunologically efficient in reducing the bacillary load, whereas the haphazard arrangement in lepromatous leprosy favours bacillary proliferation.[65] It is possible that this configuration might be important in the pathogenesis of sarcoidosis and other granulomatous diseases.

Patients with erythema nodosum due to sarcoidosis have a reduced percentage of OKT3 and OKT4 and a major decrease in the OKT8 suppressor subset. This indicates a defective circulating suppressor T cell activity in acute sarcoidosis with erythema nodosum.[66]

LYMPHOKINES AND MONOKINES

Lymphokines are the humoral products of antigen-stimulated sensitised T cells.

The activated macrophage, bearing cell-surface HLA-DR + gene products, when stimulated by antigen produces interleukin-1, which in turn activates OKT4 helper-inducer cells. These activated T4 cells produce interleukin-2, which then causes a tenfold clonal replication of these T4 helper cells. Interleukin-2 is a 15,000 to 20,000 dalton glycoprotein; it is the T cell growth factor that signals clonal proliferation in the lungs. It does not stimulate blood T lymphocytes.[67] The action of interleukin-1 on the T lymphocyte may call into play a prostaglandin-induced feedback mechanism that is inhibited by prostaglandin inhibitors. Interleukin-2 production is inhibited by cyclosporin A (Fig. 13–4). Several other soluble and secretory products play an important role in inhibiting macrophage migration away from the sarcoid battleground.

REFERENCES

1. James DG, Neville E, Walker AN. Immunology of sarcoidosis. Am J Med. 59:388, 1975.
2. James DG, Jones Williams W. Immunology of sarcoidosis. Am J Med. 72:5, 1982.
3. Davies BH, Jones K, Evans P, Jones Williams W, Williams JD. Thymic lymphocyte response in sarcoidosis: effect of sera and levamisole. In Jones Williams W, Davies BH (eds): Sarcoidosis. Cardiff, Alpha and Omega Press. p 477, 1980.
4. Hunninghake GW, Crystal RG. Pulmonary sarcoidosis: a disorder mediated by excess helper T-lymphocyte activity. N Engl J Med. 305:429, 1981.
5. Crystal RG, Robert WC, Hunninghake GW. Pulmonary sarcoidosis: a disease characterised and perpetuated by activated lung T-lymphocytes. Ann Intern Med. 94:73, 1981.
6. Semenzato G, Pezzutto A, Cipriani A, Gasparotto G. Imbalance of Ty and Tu lymphocyte subpopulations in patients with sarcoidosis. J Clin Lab Immunol. 4:95, 1980.
7. Semenzato G, Pezzutto A. Insights into the immunopathogenesis of sarcoidosis. Immunol Clin Sper. 1:35, 1982.
8. Semenzato G, Pezzutto A, Chilosi M, Pizzoli G. T lymphocyte distribution in the lymph nodes of sarcoidosis patients. N Engl J Med. 306:48, 1982.
9. Silverstein E, Friedland J, Stanek AE, Smith PR. Pathogenesis of sarcoidosis. Mechanism of angiotensin converting enzyme (ACE) elevation. T lymphocyte modulation of enzyme induction in mononuclear phagocytes: enzyme properties. In Chretien J, Marsac J, Saltiel JC (eds): Proc 9th Internat Conf Sarcoidosis. Paris, Pergamon Press. p 319, 1983.

10. Radermecker M, Gustin M, Saint-Remy P, Broux R, Sambon Y. Correlation between serum angiotensin-converting enzyme and bronchoalveolar lymphocytes in sarcoidosis. *In* Chretien J, Marsac J, Saltiel JC (eds): Proc 9th Internat Conf Sarcoidosis. Paris, Pergamon Press. p 634, 1983.
11. Parish RW, Williams JD, Davies BH. Serum beta-2-microglobulin and angiotensin-converting enzyme activity in sarcoidosis. Thorax. 37:936, 1982.
12. Mornex JF, Biot N, Pacheco Y, Perrin-Fayolle C, Vincent C, Revillard JP. β2 microglobulin levels in serum and bronchoalveolar lavage fluid from patients with sarcoidosis. *In* Chretien J, Marsac J, Saltiel JC (eds): Proc 9th Internat Conf Sarcoidosis. Paris, Pergamon Press. p 372, 1983.
13. Morishita M, Torii Y, Ichimura K, Takada K, Suzuki T, Ina Y, Aoki H, Sugiura T, Yamamoto M. Serum and bronchoalveolar lavage level of β2 microglobulin in patients with sarcoidosis. *In* Chretien J, Marsac J, Saltiel JC (eds): Proc 9th Internat Conf Sarcoidosis. Paris, Pergamon Press. p 383, 1983.
14. Pezzutto A, Fagiolo U, Corsano A, Cappellotto I, Volpato C, Agostini C, Cipriani A, Semenzato G. Ia-like antigens of T lymphocytes in active and inactive sarcoidosis. *In* Chretien J, Marsac J, Saltiel JC (eds): Proc 9th Internat Conf Sarcoidosis. Paris, Pergamon Press. p 162, 1983.
15. Jones Williams W. Activated mononuclear cells. *In* Cumming G, Bonsignore G (eds): Cellular Biology of the Lung. New York, Plenum Press. p 175, 1982.
16. Rossi AG, Hunninghake GW, Crystal RG. Evaluation of inflammatory and immune processes in the interstitial lung disorders: use of bronchoalveolar lavage. *In* Cumming G, Bonsignore G (eds): Cellular Biology of the Lung. New York, Plenum Press. p 107, 1982.
17. Kanegasaki S, Homma YJ, Washikazi M, Homma H. Chemoluminescence response of mononuclear phagocytes from patients with sarcoidosis and other granulomatous disorders. *In* Chretien J, Marsac J, Saltiel JC (eds): Proc 9th Internat Conf Sarcoidosis. Paris, Pergamon Press. p 600, 1983.
18. Goodwin JS, Webb DR. Regulations of the immune response by prostaglandins. Clin Immunol Immunopathol. 15:106, 1980.
19. James EMV, Jones Williams W. Fine structure and histochemistry of epithelioid cells in sarcoidosis. Thorax. 29:115, 1974.
20. Eckert H, Christ R, Rotte KH. Morphological parameters for the estimation of clinical course and prognosis in sarcoidosis. *In* Chretien J, Marsac J, Saltiel JC (eds): Proc 9th Internat Conf Sarcoidosis. Paris, Pergamon Press. p 649, 1983.
21. Ina Y, Yamamoto M, Takada K, Sigiura T, Morishita M, Aoki B, Torii Y, Ichimura K, Suzuki T, Yoshikawa K. Killer and natural killer activities in patients with sarcoidosis. *In* Chretien J, Marsac J, Saltiel JC (eds): Proc 9th Internat Conf Sarcoidosis. Paris, Pergamon Press. p 168, 1983.
22. Tracey DE. The requirement of macrophages in the augmentation of natural killer cell activity by BCG. J Immunol. 123:840, 1979.
23. Yoneda T, Kasai M, Ishibashi J, Nishikawa K, Tokunaga T, Mikami R. Natural killer cell activity in pulmonary tuberculosis. Br J Dis Chest. 77:185, 1983.
24. Romer FK, Solling K, Solling J. Free light chains of immunoglobulins, angiotensin-converting enzyme and circulating immune complexes in sarcoidosis. *In* Chretien J, Marsac J, Saltiel JC (eds): Proc 9th Internat Conf Sarcoidosis. Paris, Pergamon Press. p 178, 1983.
25. Williams JD, Davies BH, Jones Williams W. Personal series (unpublished).
26. Biot N, Harf R, Pacheco Y, Perrin-Fayolle M. Protein markers of inflammation in sarcoidosis (BAL fluid and serum). *In* Chretien J, Marsac J, Saltiel JC (eds): Proc 9th Internat Conf Sarcoidosis. Paris, Pergamon Press. p 645, 1983.
27. Buneaux JJ, Leclerc P, Lebeau LE, Gosselin H, Buneaux F. Relationship between the levels of protein and enzymes in serum and in bronchoalveolar lavage liquid in the case of sarcoidosis. *In* Chretien J, Marsac J, Saltiel JC (eds): Proc 9th Internat Conf Sarcoidosis. Paris, Pergamon Press. p 645, 1983.
28. Fagerhol MD, Dale I, Anderson T. Release quantitation of a leucocyte-derived protein. Scand J Haematol. 24:393, 1980.
29. Stanislav-Leguern G, Leclerc P, Baumann F Ch, Mordelet-Dambrine M, Huchon G, Andreux JP, Marsac J, Rochemaure J, Chretien J. Angiotensin-converting enzyme in bronchoalveolar fluid serum as indicators of spread of untreated sarcoidosis. *In* Chretien J, Marsac J, Saltiel JC (eds): Proc 9th Internat Conf Sarcoidosis. Paris, Pergamon Press. p 356, 1983.
30. Haslam PL, Coutts II, Watling AF, Cromwell O, Du Bois RM, Townsend PJ, Collins JY,

Turner-Warwick M. Bronchoalveolar lavage features associated with radiographic evidence of fibrosis in pulmonary sarcoidosis. *In* Chretien J, Marsac J, Saltiel JC (eds): Proc 9th Internat Conf Sarcoidosis. Paris, Pergamon Press. p 209, 1983.

31. Hedfors E. Immunological aspects of sarcoidosis. Scand J Resp Dis. 56:1, 1975.
32. Daniele RP, McMillan LJ, Danker JH, Rossman MD. Immune complexes in sarcoidosis: a correlation with activity and duration of disease. Chest. 261:74, 1978.
33. Saint-Remy JM, Mitchell DN, Cole PJ. Variations in immunoglobulin levels and circulating immune complexes in sarcoidosis: correlation with extent of disease and duration of symptoms. *In* Chretien, J, Marsac J, Saltiel JC (eds): Proc 9th Internat Conf Sarcoidosis. Paris, Pergamon Press. p 596, 1982.
34. Glikmann G, Nillsen H, Pallingaard G, Christensen KM, Svehag SE. Circulating immuno-complexes, free antigen and alpha 2 anti trypsin levels in sarcoidosis patients. Scand J Resp Dis. 60:317, 1979.
35. Gupta PG, Knepars F, DeRemee RA, Huston KA, McDuffie FC. Pulmonary and extrapulmonary sarcoidosis in relation to circulating immune complexes. A quantification of immune complexes by two radioimmunoassays. Ann Resp Dis. 116:261, 1977.
36. Rottoli L, Rottoli P. Immune complexes in sarcoidosis. *In* Lenzini L, Rottoli P (eds): La Sarcoidosi. Sienna, Centro Stampa Universita. p 405, 1981.
37. Selroos O, Klockars M, Kekomak R, Pentinnen K, Lindström P, Wager O. Circulating immune complexes in sarcoidosis. Acta Immunol Scand. 3:129, 1980.
38. Ghose T, Landrigan P, Asif A. Localisation of immunoglobulin and complement in pulmonary sarcoid granulomas. Chest. 66:264, 1974.
39. Fox B, Sousha S, Jamesk R, Miller GC. Immune histological study of human lungs by immunoperoxidase technique. J Clin Pathol. 35:144, 1982.
40. Ridley MJ, Marianaygam Y, Spector WG. Experimental granulomas included by mycobacterial immune complexes in rats. J Pathol. 136:59, 1982.
41. Tomasi TB. Serum factors which suppress the immune response. Regulatory mechanisms in lymphocyte activation. *In* Lucas DO (ed): Proc 11th Leucocyte Conf. Arizona, Academic Press. p 219, 1976.
42. Voorting-Hawking M, Michael JG. Isolation and characterisation of immunoregulatory factors from normal human serum. J Immunol. 118:505, 1977.
43. Shima K, Ikeda S, Horinchi S, Tsuda T, Tokuomi H. The influence of sarcoid serum on normal T lymphocyte. *In* Jones Williams W, Davies BH (eds): Sarcoidosis. Cardiff, Alpha and Omega Press. p 459, 1980.
44. Mangi RJ, Dwyer JM, Kantor FS. The effects of plasma upon lymphocyte response in-vitro demonstration of a humoral inhibitor in patients with sarcoidosis. Clin Exp Immunol. 18:519, 1974.
45. Semenzato G, Cipriani A, Golombati M, Amadori G, Gasparotto G, Serembe M. Inhibitors of T cell immune function in sarcoidosis. *In* Jones Williams W, Davies BH (eds): Sarcoidosis. Cardiff, Alpha and Omega Press. p 466, 1980.
46. Semenzato G, Pezzuto A, Agostini C, Gasparotto G, Cipriani A. Immunoregulation in sarcoidosis. Clin Immunol Immunopathol. 19:416, 1981.
47. Moretta L, Moretta A, Canonica GW, Bacigalupo A, Mingari MC, Cerottini JC. Receptors for immunoglobulins on resting and activated T lymphocytes. Immunol Rev. 56:141, 1981.
48. Davies BH, Williams JD, Smith M, Jones Williams W, Jones K. Peripheral blood lymphocytes in sarcoidosis. Pathol Res Pract. 175:97, 1982.
49. James DG, Neville E, Siltzbach LE, Turiaf J, Battesti JP, Sharma OP, Hosoda Y, Mikami R, Odaka M, Villar TG, Djuric B, Douglas AC, Middleton W, Karlish A, Blasi A, Olivieri D, Press P. A worldwide review of sarcoidosis. Ann NY Acad Sci. 278:321, 1976.
50. Hardt F, Wanstrup J. Sarcoidosis. An "in vitro" Kveim reaction based on the leucocyte migration test. Acta Path Microbiol Scand. 76:493, 1969.
51. Jones Williams W, Pioli E, Jones DJ, Calcraft B, Johnson AJ, Dighero H. In vitro Kveim-induced macrophage inhibition factor KMIF test in sarcoidosis, Crohn's disease and tuberculosis. *In* Iwai K, Hosoda Y (eds): Proc 6th Internat Conf Sarcoidosis. Tokyo, Univ. Press. p 44, 1974.
52. Topilsky M, Williams N, Siltzbach LE, Glade PG. Lymphocytic responses in sarcoidosis. Lancet 1:117, 1975.
53. Hardt F, Veien N, Bendixen G, Brodthagen H, Faber Y, Genner J, Heckscher T, Ringsted J, Freiesleben S, Sørensen J, Wanstrup J, Wiik A. Immunological studies in sarcoidosis. A comparison of in vivo and in vitro Kveim tests. Ann N Y Acad Sci. 278:711, 1976.

54. Horsmanheimo M, Horsmanheimo A, Fudenberg HH, Siltzbach LE, McKee KT. Kveim test reactivity with leukocyte migration in agarose and lymphocytic transformation tests. *In* Jones Williams W, Davies BH (eds): Sarcoidosis. Cardiff, Alpha and Omega Press. p 186, 1980.
55. Cohn ZA, Fedorko ME, Hirsch JG, Morse SI, Siltzbach LE. The distribution of Kveim activity in subcellular fractions from sarcoid lymph nodes. *In* Turiaf J, Chabot J, James DG, Zatouroff M (eds): La Sarkoidose. Paris, Masson and Co. p 141, 1967.
56. Chase MW, Siltzbach LE. Concentration of the active principle responsible for the Kveim reaction. *In* Turiaf J, Chabot J, James DG, Zatouroff M (eds): La Sarkoidose. Paris, Masson and Co. p 150, 1967.
57. Middleton WG, Douglas AC. Further experience with Edinburgh prepared Kveim-Siltzbach test suspension. *In* Jones Williams W, Davies BH (eds): Sarcoidosis. Cardiff, Alpha and Omega Press. p 655, 1980.
58. Bradstreet CMP, Dighero MW, Mitchell DN. The Kveim test: analysis of results of tests using K19 materials. *In* Jones Williams W, Davies BH (eds): Sarcoidosis. Cardiff, Alpha and Omega Press. p 674, 1980.
59. Neville E, James DG, Brewerton DA, James DCO, Cockburn C, Fenichal B. HLA antigens and clinical features of sarcoidosis. *In* Jones Williams W, Davies BH (eds): Sarcoidosis. Cardiff, Alpha and Omega Press. p 201, 1980.
60. Gardner J, Kennedy HG, Hamblin A, Jones E. HLA associations in sarcoidosis: a study of two ethnic groups. Thorax. 39:19, 1984.
61. Turton CWG, Turner-Warwick M, Morris L, Lawler SD. HLA in familial sarcoidosis. *In* Jones Williams W, Davies BH (eds): Sarcoidosis. Cardiff, Alpha and Omega Press. p 195, 1980.
62. Al-Arif L, Goldstein RA, Affronti LF, Janicki BW, Foellmer JW. HLA antigens and sarcoidosis in a North American black population. *In* Jones Williams W, Davies BH (eds): Sarcoidosis. Cardiff, Alpha and Omega Press. p 206, 1980.
63. Newill CA, Johns CJ, Cohen BH, Diamond EL, Bias WB. Sarcoidosis HLA and immunoglobulin markers in Baltimore blacks. *In* Chretien J, Marsac J, Saltiel JC (eds): Proc 9th Internat Conf Sarcoidosis. Paris, Pergamon Press. p 253, 1983.
64. Mishra BB, Poulter LW, Janossy G, James DG. The distribution of lymphoid- and macrophage-like cell subsets of sarcoid and Kveim granulomata; possible mechanism of negative PPD reaction in sarcoidosis. Clin Exp Immunol. 54:705, 1983.
65. Modlin RL, Hofman FM, Meyer PR, Sharma OP, Taylor CR, Rea TH. In situ demonstration of T lymphocyte subsets in granulomatous inflammation: leprosy, rhinoscleroma and sarcoidosis. Clin Exp Immunol. 51:430, 1983.
66. Faure M, Nicolas JF, Gaucherard M, Czernicielewski J, Mauduit G, Thivolet J. Numeration of T cell subsets in sarcoidosis using monoclonal antibodies; decreased levels of peripheral blood T cells and cells with suppressor T cell phenotype. Dermatologica 165:88, 1982.
67. Pinkston P, Bitterman B, Crystal RG. Spontaneous release of interleukin-2 by lung T lymphocytes in active pulmonary sarcoidosis. N Engl J Med. 308:793, 1983.

14

Criteria of Activity

During the last 100 years, there were very few markers of activity of sarcoidosis or criteria of cure. During the last 10 years, we have been inundated with fresh markers of activity, so many that it is becoming difficult to choose the most helpful (Table 14–1). We have grouped them as follows: (1) clinical features that indicate activity and bedside techniques that proclaim activity, (2) biochemical markers, (3) immunological markers, and (4) other markers.

CLINICAL AND BEDSIDE TECHNIQUES

Erythema nodosum, uveitis, and maculopapular eruptions point to active disease. If posterior uveitis is suspected, then *fluorescein angiography* provides the new dimension of leakage of dye, indicating retinal vasculitis. Other clinical features of activity are dactylitis, polyarthralgia, myopathy, neuropathy, granulomatous scars, splenomegaly, lymphadenopathy, and enlargement of salivary and lacrimal glands.

There is no single *chest radiograph* that can be interpreted as a sign of activity, but changing chest x-ray abnormalities emphasise activity.

The electrocardiogram is not helpful in assessing activity, but a 24-hour ECG tape may reveal cardiac arrythmias due to sarcoidosis.

LUNG FUNCTION

The single-breath diffusing capacity (transfer factor) and particularly the exercise KCO are helpful lung function tests. In the earliest stage of hilar adenopathy there is reduction in transfer factor and arterial oxygen tension. With pulmonary infiltration there is a reduction of vital capacity, airway resistance, maximum mid-expiratory flow, and arterial oxygen tension on exercise. These tests, however, are unhelpful in predicting the course of the disease.[1]

192

Table 14–1. Markers of Activity of Sarcoidosis

Clinical*	Biochemical†	Immunological‡
Erythema nodosum	Hypercalcaemia	T cell
		Helper/suppressor ratio
Uveitis	Hypercalciuria	Lung
		Blood
Maculopapular rash	SACE	Tissues
Dactylitis	LACE	Interleukin-2
Polyarthralgia	Lysozyme	Ia cells
Myopathy	β glucuronidase	K and NK cells
Neuropathy	Fibronectin	B cells
		Immunoglobulins
Granulomatous scars	Urinary hydroxyproline	IgG, IgA
		Free light chains
Splenomegaly		
		Immune complexes
Lymphadenopathy		
		Skin tests
Salivary and lacrimal gland		Tuberculin
enlargement		Kveim-Siltzbach
Cardiac arrhythmia		
		Others
Changing chest x-ray		
Changing lung function		Radioactive gallium scan
Fluorescein angiography		Thallium-201 myocardial scan
		Fresh granulomas

*See relevant chapters.
†See Chapter 12.
‡See Chapter 13.

BIOCHEMICAL MARKERS (see Chapter 12)

Hypercalcaemia and hypercalciuria have long been recognized as indices of activity. They are transient in acute disease but persistent and more serious in chronic, longstanding disease and may lead to nephrocalcinosis.

Both serum (SACE) and lavage (LACE) angiotensin-converting enzyme levels are good indices of activity and extent of the disease. In a collaboratory study of 1,070 patients with 12 centres in 6 countries, SACE and LACE levels were compared with radiological staging with similar results from all the centres.[2] SACE levels were raised in 27 per cent of patients in Stage 0, 56 per cent of those in Stage 1, 72 per cent of those in Stage 2, and 56 per cent of those in Stage 3. A significant difference between Stage 2 patients and those in other stages is well brought out in Stage 2 patients with clinical extrathoracic dissemination as compared with Stage 1 patients without this dissemination.[3] LACE levels also follow the same pattern, with the best correlation between SACE and LACE levels seen in intrathoracic rather than extrathoracic patients.[4] As epithelioid cells are a source of SACE,[5] these and other findings emphasise that active granulomas are still present in radiological Stage 3 cases.

SACE levels correlate with a number of other markers of disease activity (Table 14–2). There is a good correlation between macrophage-derived enzymes and serum lysozyme,[6, 7] β-glucuronidase,[7] and fibronectin[8] in lavage fluid, numbers and activity of T cells in lavage fluid,[9] numbers of killer lymphocytes in the circulation,[10] radioactive gallium uptake,[11] and the Kveim-Siltzbach test.[12] Romer[13] has shown an interesting correlation between SACE and hypercalcaemia and feels that a rise in both distinguishes the hypercalcaemia of sarcoidosis from that of non-sarcoid patients.

SACE levels show no definite correlation with levels of serum immunoglobulins, free light chains and circulating immune complexes,[14] β_2 microglobulin,[15] sedimentation rate, tuberculin skin reactivity, and levels of collagenase and elastase in lavage fluid.

Raised levels of polymorph/macrophage-derived enzymes (lysozyme and β-glucuronidase) alone are of marginal value in judging disease activity. Increased lysozyme levels have been demonstrated in both sarcoid serum and lymph nodes of sarcoid patients,[16] but, as noted previously, raised serum levels are of most value when combined with raised SACE levels.[6] This is also true of β-glucuronidase.

Measurement of factors concerned with collagen formation and degradation is also partly related to activity. Fibronectin levels are increased in the lavage fluid of patients with enhanced macrophage activity.[8] The role of proteolytic collagenase and elastase may be important in the formation of auto-immune antigens inducing fibrosis (see Chapter 3). It is not yet proven whether these and other macrophage-induced fibroblast growth-promoting factors correlate with histological evidence of increasing fibrosis. Measurements of collagen breakdown products in urine, by determining hydroxyproline levels, have suggested that raised levels relate to activity with a fall in burnt-out fibrotic disease.[17]

IMMUNOLOGICAL MARKERS (see Chapter 13)

There is redistribution of T helper (OKT4) cells to the sites of maximal activity, with a predominance of T suppressor (OKT8) cells in the peripheral blood.[18] It appears that in addition to pooling in the lungs, T4 produces

Table 14–2. Tests That Either Do or Do Not Correlate with SACE

Positive Significant Correlation	No Significant Correlation
Serum lysozyme	Serum immunoglobulins
Fibronectin	Free light chains
β-glucuronidase	Immune complexes
Pulmonary T-lymphocyte activity	Serum β_2 microglobulins
Circulating K and NK activity	Sedimentation rate
Radioactive gallium uptake	Tuberculin skin test
Kveim-Siltzbach skin test	Collagenase
Sarcoid hypercalcaemia	Elastase
Chest x-ray resolution	

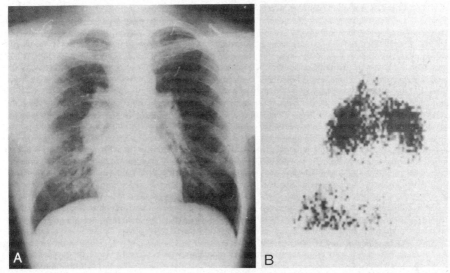

Figure 14–1. Radioactive gallium scan showing uptake by (A) bilateral sarcoid hilar lymph nodes and (B) normal liver. (Courtesy of Dr. Gianfranco Rizzato, Milan.)

interleukin-2, leading to local excess production of the same cell[19] (see Fig. 13–3).

B cell markers include an excess of free light chain radicals in active disease[14] and IgG and IgA in lavage fluid in progressive disease.[20]

Levels of immune complexes are only doubtfully increased in active as compared with chronic disease, for results from various groups disagree.

The easily performed tuberculin and Kveim-Siltzbach skin tests are of some value in determining activity. In longstanding fibrotic disease the negative tuberculin test may become weakly positive and the Kveim-Siltzbach test negative.

RADIOACTIVE SCANS

Gallium Scanning

The activated macrophages of sarcoid tissue avidly accumulate gallium and may be used for delineating active granulomas. It is also taken up by protein of inflammatory exudate. Three days following an intravenous injection of 3 mCi of Ga^{67} citrate, simultaneous anterior and posterior scans of the entire thorax are done.[11, 21, 22] As steroids suppress gallium uptake, it is advisable to stop treatment for about one week before performing the test.[22] Active sarcoid tissue accumulates gallium, and this technique helps to distinguish sarcoid hilar lymph nodes from pulmonary arteries (Fig. 14–1), parenchymal granulomas from other pulmonary infiltrates, and granulomas from hyaline fibrosis. Gallium is taken up by liver, spleen, and bone in the normal person, so it does not help to detect granulomas in the abdominal

Table 14–3. Tissue and Serological Markers in Sarcoidosis

Cells and Markers	Tissue	Blood/Serum Markers	Bronchopulmonary Lavage
Tm (helper)		Normal	High (twice blood level)
Tg (suppressor)		High	Low
T4:T8	Normal	0.8:1	10.5:1
IaT cells		Increased	
		Increased levels of β_2 microglobulins	
Killer cells K, NK		Increased antibody production, particularly advanced pulmonary disease	
B cells	Inconspicuous	Not elevated	Not elevated
Immunoglobulins	Present	Increased	Increased
Kappa and lambda light chains		Increased, particularly chronic active disease	
Macrophage	Prominent		Low (active disease)
			High (inactive disease)
Gallium uptake	Increased		
ACE	Present	Increased	Increased
Lysozyme		Increased	Increased
Collagenase		Increased	Increased
Lysosomal enzymes	Increased	Possible increase	

viscera or the nervous system. Liver uptake should be regarded as the control, and lung uptake is measured by comparison with the density of liver uptake. It should not be forgotten that this test is not specific for sarcoidosis; uptake is noted in asbestosis, silicosis, fibrosing alveolitis, cancer, and bleomycin lung and in lymphomas. Based on a variety of clinical, radiological, and lavage findings and criteria of activity with ACE estimations, gallium scanning is probably more accurate than chest radiography.[11, 12, 22] A recent international survey* showed that 29.5 per cent (39/132) of untreated patients with radiological State 0 (normal chest radiography) showed Ga[67] uptake in pulmonary and/or mediastinal glands.

Radioactive thallium-201 is taken up by myocardial sarcoid tissue and by the ischaemic myocardium. Exercise gets rid of radioactive thallium from myocardium sarcoid tisue but not from areas of ischaemia.[23]

OTHER PARAMETERS

Detailed analysis of the cellular content of granulomas has shown that "fresh," non-fibrous granulomas are a feature of recent active disease (see Chapter 3). Electron microscopy studies suggest that, in sarcoid granulomas, early epithelioid cells are rich in endoplasmic reticulum compared with more

---

*G. Rizzato, personal communication.

mature cells, which are rich in secretory vessicles.[24] This was confirmed in experimental BCG-induced granulomas, including cell markers.[25] Recent identification of distribution of T subsets and macrophages in (early) Kveim-Siltzbach skin biopsies[26] with new techniques including immunochemistry and histocytochemistry may lead to the identification of other cell markers and may allow us to differentiate active, quiescent, and fibrosing granulomas (Table 14–3).

REFERENCES

1. Sears MR. Pulmonary gas transfer and alveolar-arterial oxygen difference in sarcidosis. *In* Jones Williams W, Davies BH (eds): Sarcoidosis. Cardiff, Alpha and Omega Press. p 343, 1980.
2. Studdy PR, James DG. The specificity and sensitivity of serum angiotensin-converting enzymes in sarcoidosis and other diseases. Experience in twelve centres in six different countries. *In* Chretien J, Marsac J, Saltiel JC (eds): Proc 9th Internat Conf Sarcoidosis. Paris, Pergamon Press. p 332, 1983.
3. Sandron D, Lecossier D, Grodet A, Barbe C, Basset G, Battesti JP. Serum angiotensin converting enzyme (SACE) and the diffusion of the sarcoid granuloma, evolution and therapeutic interest. *In* Chretien J, Marsac J, Saltiel JC (eds): Proc 9th Internat Conf Sarcoidosis. Paris, Pergamon Press. p 345, 1983.
4. Stanislas-Leguern G, Leclerc P, Baumann FC, Mordelet-Dambrine M, Huchon GJ, Andreux JP, Marsac J, Rochemaure J, Chretien J. Angiotensin converting enzyme in bronchoalveolar fluid and serum as indicators of spread of untreated sarcoidosis. *In* Chretien J, Marsac J, Saltiel JC (eds): Proc 9th Internat Conf Sarcoidosis. Paris, Pergamon. p 356, 1983.
5. Silverstein E, Friedland J, Stanek AE, Smith PR, Deason DR, Lyons HA. Pathogenesis of sarcoidosis. Mechanism of angiotensin converting enzyme elevation: T-lymphocyte modulation of enzyme induction in mononclear phagocytes; enzyme properties. *In* Chretien J, Marsac J, Saltiel JC (eds): Proc 9th Internat Conf Sarcoidosis. Paris, Pergamon Press. p 319, 1983.
6. Selroos O, Tiitien H, Gronhagen-Riska F, Fyhrquist F, Klockars M. Angiotensin converting enzyme and lysozyme in sarcoidosis. *In* Jones Williams W, Davies BH (eds): Sarcoidosis. Cardiff, Alpha and Omega Press. p 303, 1980.
7. Shigematsu M, Matsuba K, Taira M, Hirose N, Koga T. Elevated serum angiotensin converting enzyme in sarcoidosis and renal disorders. *In* Chretien J, Marsac J, Saltiel JC (eds): Proc 9th Internat Conf Sarcoidosis. Paris, Pergamon Press. p 637, 1983.
8. Rennard SI, Hunninghake GW, Bitterman PB, Crystal RG. Production of fibronectin by the human alveolar macrophage, a mechanism for the recruitment of fibroblast to sites of tissue injury in the interstitial lung diseases. Proc Natl Acad Sci. 78:7147, 1981.
9. Radermecker M, Gustin M, Saint-Remy P, Broux R, Sambon Y. Correlation between serum angiotensin converting enzyme and bronchoalveolar lymphocytes in sarcoidosis. *In* Chretien J, Marsac J, Saltiel JC (eds): Proc 9th Internat Conf Sarcoidosis. Paris, Pergamon Press. p 634, 1983.
10. Ina Y, Yamamoto M, Takada K, Sugiura T, Muramatsu M, Morishita M, Aoki H, Torii Y, Ichimura K, Yoshikawa K, Suzuki M. Killer and natural killer activities in patients with sarcoidosis. *In* Chretien J, Marsac J, Saltiel JC (eds). Proc 9th Internat Conf Sarcoidosis. Paris, Pergamon Press, p 168, 1983.
11. Nosal A, Schleissner LA, Mishkin FS, Lieberman J. Angiotensin converting enzymes and Gallium scan in non-invasive evaluation of sarcoidosis. Ann Intern Med. 90:328, 1979.
12. Siltzbach LE, Krakoff L, Dorph D, Tierstein AS. Elevated levels of serum angiotensin converting enzyme (kinase 11) and lysozyme levels in sarcoidosis. *In* Jones Williams W, Davies BH (eds): Sarcoidosis. Cardiff, Alpha and Omega Press. p 298, 1980.
13. Romer FK. S-angiotensin converting enzyme (SACE) in hypercalcaemia due to sarcoidosis and other disorders. *In* Chretien J, Marsac J, Saltiel JC (eds): Proc 9th Internat Conf Sarcoidosis. Paris, Pergamon Press. p 637, 1983.

14. Romer FK, Solling K, Solling J. Free light chains of immunoglobulin, angiotensin-converting enzyme, and circulating immune complexes in sarcoidosis. *In* Chretien J, Marsac J, Saltiel JC (eds): Proc 9th Internat Conf Sarcoidosis. Paris, Pergamon Press. p 178, 1983.
15. Parish RW, Williams JD, Davies BH. Serum β_2 immunoglobulin and angiotensin-converting enzyme activity in sarcoidosis. Thorax. 37:936, 1982.
16. Silverstein E, Friedland J, Lyons HA, Gourin A. Elevation of angiotensin converting enzyme in granulomatous lymph nodes and serum in sarcoidosis; clinical and possible pathogenic significance. Ann NY Acad Sci. 278:498, 1976.
17. Massaro D, Handler AE, Katz S, Yound RC. Excretion of hydroxyproline in patients with sarcoidosis. Am Rev Resp Dis. 93:929, 1966.
18. Crystal RG, Hunninghake GW, Gadek JE, Keogh BA, Rennard SJ, Bitterman PB. The pathogenesis of sarcoidosis. *In* Chretien J, Marsac J, Saltiel JC (eds): Proc 9th Internat Conf Sarcoidosis. Paris, Pergamon Press. p 13, 1983.
19. Pinkston P, Bitterman PB, Crystal RG. Spontaneous release of interleukin-2 by lung T lymphocytes in active pulmonary sarcoidosis. N Engl J Med. 308:793, 1983.
20. Saint-Remy R, Mitchell D, Cole J. Variation in immunoglobulin levels and circulating immune complexes in sarcoidosis: correlation with extent of disease and duration of symptoms. *In* Chretien J, Marsac J, Saltiel JC (eds): Proc 9th Internat Conf Sarcoidosis. Paris, Pergamon Press. p 596, 1983.
21. Hoffer P. Gallium mechanism. J Nucl Med. 21:282, 1980.
22. Klech H, Kohn H, Kummer P, Mostbeck A. Value of different parameters for the assessment of activity in sarcoidosis: X-ray, Gallium scanning, serum-ACE levels and blood lymphocyte subpopulation. *In* Chretien J, Marsac J, Saltiel JC (eds): Proc 9th Internat Conf Sarcoidosis. Paris, Pergamon Press. p 389, 1983.
23. Sharma OP. Thallium-201 imaging in the management of mycardial sarcoidosis. *In* Chretien J, Marsac J, Saltiel JC (eds): Proc 9th Internat Conf Sarcoidosis. Paris, Pergamon Press. p 619, 1983.
24. James EMV, Jones Williams W. Fine structure and histochemistry of epithelioid cells in sarcoidosis. Thorax. 29:115, 1974.
25. Williams GT. Functional studies and surface receptor characteristics of isolated epithelioid cells from experimental granulomas. *In* Chretien J, Marsac J, Saltiel JC (eds): Proc 9th Internat Conf Sarcoidosis. Paris, Pergamon Press. p 76, 1983.
26. Mishra BB, Poulter LW, Janossy G, James DG. The distribution of macrophage and lymphocyte subsets in the sarcoid and Kveim test granulomas suggests the pathogenesis of the negative PPD reaction in sarcoidosis. Clin Exp Immunol. 54:705, 1983.

15

Differential Diagnosis

We have presented a classification of granulomatous disorders (see Table 2–1) to indicate that sarcoidosis is but one member of a large family of similar disorders. When confronted with a granulomatous disease we do not automatically go through all the list, but in a difficult, problem patient it is as well to be reminded that sarcoidosis has numerous mimics and is reminiscent of syphilis in the pre-penicillin era.

The differential diagnosis demands a synthesis of information provided by the clinician, radiologist, histologist, microbiologist, and chemical pathologist. Sometimes he may be one and the same person. Since this is how the differential diagnosis is made in practice, we have used a joint clinicopathological approach.

INFECTIONS

Exclusion of pathogenic organisms is done by special stains, culture, and serum antibody titres when applicable. This is particularly necessary in certain endemic areas or in immigrant populations harbouring tuberculosis, leprosy, bilharziasis, and helminthiasis.

Infective Agents (Table 15–1)

Fungi

They comprise *Histoplasma*, *Coccidioides*, *Blastomyces*, *Sporothrix*, *Aspergillus*, and *Cryptococcus* spp. (Table 15–2). It is important to exclude fungal infection in all granulomatous disorders, whether localised or disseminated disease.

Protozoa

They comprise *Leishmania* and *Toxoplasma* spp.

Leishmania. The clinical forms of leishmaniasis are visceral, cutaneous, and mucocutaneous. *Leishmania donovani* causes kala-azar. Leishman-Dono-

Table 15–1. Infective Granulomas

Fungi	Mycobacteria
Histoplasma	*Mycobacterium tuberculosis*
Coccidioides	*M. leprae*
Blastomyces	*M. kansasii*
Sporothrix	*M. marinum*
Aspergillus	*M. avian*
Cryptococcus	BCG vaccine
Protozoa	**Bacteria**
Toxoplasma	*Brucella*
Leishmania	*Francisella tularensis*
	Proprioni
Metazoa	*Yersinia*
Toxocara	
Schistosoma	**Others**
	Cat-scratch disease
Spirochaetes	Lymphogranuloma
Treponema pallidum	
T. pertenue	
T. carateum	

van bodies are found within single or focal collections of macrophages in blood; in aspirates of sternal marrow, liver, or spleen; or in special culture medium. Other helpful differentiating tests are serum antibodies, grossly elevated IgG, and a skin test.

Toxoplasma. As a result of transplacental spread of a protozoon, *Toxoplasma gondii,* infants may be stillborn or may be born with choroidoretinitis, hydrocephalus, microcephaly, encephalomyelitis, hepatosplenomegaly, or neonatal jaundice or may later develop cerebral calcification. Acute focal choroiditis in a young adult represents later relapses of congenital toxoplasmosis. Serum antibodies are positive in low titre.

Acquired toxoplasmosis presents as glandular fever. Lymph node biopsy discloses compact follicles of sarcoid tissue, and acute toxoplasmosis may be mistakenly diagnosed as sarcoidosis. Serum antibodies are present in high titre with significant rises and falls. Encephalitis in the immunodeficient may not have this antibody response.[1]

Metazoa

Toxocara and *Schistosoma* spp. are responsible for widespread chronic granulomatous inflammation.

Toxocara. Certain larval nematodes, particularly the dog and cat ascarids *Toxocara canis* and *T. cati,* may infect children, producing the syndrome of visceral larva migrans. Swallowed infected eggs emerge as larvae in the intestine, whence they pass to the liver, lungs, brain, and eye, producing eosinophilic granulomas in these different organs. This infestation should be particularly suspected in children with hepatomegaly or miliary granu-

Table 15–2. Features of Fungal Granulomatous Diseases Mimicking Sarcoidosis

Fungus	Mycosis	Clinical Features	Isolation	Other Tests Skin	Serum Antibodies	Treatment	Remarks
Histoplasma capsulatum	Histoplasmosis	*ACUTE:* erythema nodosum, "flu", pneumonia *CHRONIC:* hepatosplenomegaly, cavities (in lungs), calcification (in lungs), choroidoretinitis	Budding fungus cells within reticulo-endothelial system	+	+	Amphotericin B Ketoconazole	Endemic in Ohio, Eastern Canada, South America, Africa, S.E. Asia
Coccidioides immitis	Coccidioidomycosis	Erythema nodosum Abscess in lung, pleura, bone. Meningitis	Sporangia filled with endospores from clinical specimens	+	+	Amphotericin B Ketoconazole	Uncontrolled progressive disease, particularly in non-Caucasians More frequent in men
Blastomyces dermatitidis	Blastomycosis	Granulomata in skin, bones, prostate, epididymis	5- to 20-µm thick-walled cell in clinical specimens		+	Amphotericin B Hydroxystilbamidine	Endemic in Central and Eastern USA and Canada
Sporothrix schenkii	Sporotrichosis	Hard, non-tender subcutaneous nodule ulcerates and disseminates widely	From nodules	+		Potassium iodide Amphotericin B Miconazole	Worldwide Handlers of soil, plants, and decaying wood infected by pricking skin
Aspergillus fumigatus	Aspergillosis	Chronic bronchopulmonary abscesses Fungus balls Bronchocentric granulomatosis	Branched, septate hyphae in sputum and tissue		+	Amphotericin B Flucytosine Rifampicin Ketoconazole	Invasive form of disease in immunodeficient patients
Cryptococcus neoformans	Cryptococcosis	Pulmonary disease may disseminate, causing meningitis	Budding, encapsulated yeast in spinal fluid and sputum			Amphotericin B Flucytosine	

lomas in liver biopsies, miliary lung mottling, eosinophilia, and focal posterior uveitis or endophthalmitis, which sometimes resembles retinoblastoma. Examination of the faeces is unhelpful, since the intestinal larvae do not produce eggs. Blood and skin tests have been developed, but cross reactions may occur with other helminths.

Schistosoma. Ova are embedded within an epithelioid cell granuloma. Giant cells are of multinucleate type, and eosinophils are conspicuous. In a late stage calcified ova may be buried in fibrous nodules; they are distinguished from Schaumann's bodies because they lack the aggregated spherules and crystalline material. The immune mechanisms responsible for the schistosoma granuloma are well-recognised manifestations of cell-mediated immunity, including migration-inhibitory and eosinophilotactic factors.[2]

S. mansoni causes intestinal schistosomiasis, with portal hypertension; *S. haematobium* gives rise to vesical schistosomiasis; and *S. japonicum* is an important cause of Asian intestinal schistosomiasis.

Spirochaetes

They comprise *Treponema pallidum,* which is responsible for syphilis; *T. pertenue,* which causes jaws; and *T. carateum,* the causal agent of nonvenereal pinta in Latin America. All three disorders are chronic granulomatous disorders that may cause diagnostic confusion, particularly when there is generalised lymphadenopathy due to secondary syphilis. The distinguishing features from sarcoidosis are the excess of plasma cells, paucity of giant cells, and lack of necrosis. However, if the patient has suffered the Jarisch-Herxheimer reaction, then necrosis is evident and may resemble caseating tuberculosis.

Mycobacteria

This large group comprises *Mycobacterium tuberculosis, M. leprae,* several opportunistic mycobacteria, and BCG vaccine.

Mycobacterium tuberculosis. This is one of the most frequent causes of an infective granulomatous process (Table 15–3). The hallmark is the large central area of caseation. In patients with good resistance against the organism, the granulomas remain discrete and non-caseating and may be indistinguishable from those seen in sarcoidosis. Presumably, the macrophage–T lymphocyte partnership is efficient and well organised in its disposal of the causative organism. Under these circumstances, it is essential to attempt to detect the organism by special staining and culture. All clinical specimens labelled sarcoidosis must be cultured for mycobacteria and care taken to adjust culture temperatures to meet the requirements of various mycobacteria.

Table 15–3. Differences between Tuberculosis and Sarcoidosis

Features	Tuberculosis	Sarcoidosis
Ethnic Group	Pakistani/Indian/ Bangladeshi	West Indian/Irish
Age Incidence (Years)	Over 50	20–50
Fever	Common	Rare
Erythema Nodosum	Uncommon	Common
Uveitis		
Skin Involvement ⎫ Enlarged Parotids ⎬ Bone Cysts ⎭	Very rare	Common
Ulceration and Sinuses	Common	No
Involvement of: Pleura ⎫ Peritoneum ⎪ Pericardium ⎬ Meninges ⎪ Small Intestine ⎭	Common	Very rare
Caseation	Maximal	Minimal
Acid-Fast Bacilli	Present	Absent
Tuberculin Test	Positive in most	Negative in 65%
Kveim-Siltzbach Test	Negative	Positive in 80%
Hypercalcaemia	No	Yes
Hypercalciuria	No	Yes
Serum Angiotensin- Converting Enzyme	Elevated in up to 10%	Elevated in 60%
Calcification	Yes	Rare
Hilar Lymphadenopathy	Unilateral	Bilateral
Pulmonary Cavities	Common, early	Rare, late
Ghon Focus	Yes	No
Corticosteroids	Harmful alone	Helpful
Antituberculous Drugs	Treatment of choice	Unhelpful
Worldwide Epidemiology	Shrinking	More evident

Mycobacterium balnei. This organism, which causes "swimming-pool granuloma," infects the skin and draining axillary and inguinal lymph nodes. Although the primary skin infection may be inconspicuous, the draining lymph nodes are extensively involved and caseous. A similar microscopic picture, with conspicuous plasma cell infiltration, is noted in granulomas due to other opportunistic mycobacteria.

Mycobacterium leprae. Cell-mediated immune responses are well preserved in the localised, paucibacillary tuberculoid leprosy and difficult to demonstrate in the disseminated, multibacillary lepromatous leprosy[3] (Table 15–4).

Mononuclear phagocytes in leprosy granulomas vary from paucibacillary epithelioid cells in the tuberculoid end of the spectrum to bacilli-laden foamy macrophages in lepromatous leprosy. There is a good correlation between these macrophages and T lymphocytes. OKT4 helper-inducer cells are dispersed in close proximity to epithelioid cells in the centre of the granuloma, whereas OKT8 suppressor/cytotoxic cells are associated with interdigitating macrophages as a peripheral ring or mantle[4] in tuberculoid leprosy as in sarcoidosis (Fig. 15–1).

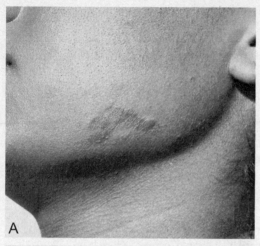

A

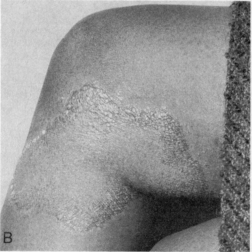

B

Figure 15–1. Tuberculoid leprosy. It resembles psoriasis clinically and histologically was identical to sarcoidosis.

Brucella

The granuloma consists of loose collections of macrophages admixed with polymorphs, plasma cells, and occasional eosinophils. The granulomas are not compact as in sarcoidosis, and Langhans-type giant cells and caseation are both inconspicuous and exceptional.

Yersinia Enterocolitis[5]

Yersinia (Pasteurella) causes granulomatous mesenteric lymphadenitis. Discrete focal granulomas are unusual. Numerous epithelioid cells are arranged around many areas of necrosis containing eosinophils and numerous polymorphs to give the picture of a pseudo-abscess. The same features are seen in the lymph nodes in *cat-scratch disease*, which may be related.

Infective granulomas may mimic sarcoidosis, so it is important, among other factors, to pay attention to the age of the patient (Table 15–5) and the environmental background (Table 15–6).

NEOPLASIA

Sarcoid granulomas related to tumours may cause diagnostic confusion. First, sarcoid granulomas may be found in various tumours and in their draining lymph nodes, particularly those draining carcinoma of the lung,

Table 15–4. Immunology of Sarcoidosis and Leprosy

Feature	Sarcoidosis	Leprosy	
		Lepromatous	*Tuberculoid*
Skin tests			
Lepromin			
Human	Negative	Negative	Positive
Armadillo		Negative	Positive
Tuberculin	Negative	Positive	Positive
Candida	Negative	Weak positive	Positive
Trichophytin	Negative	Weak positive	Positive
Kveim-Siltzbach	Positive	Negative	Negative
T Cells			Normal
Helper	Active in lungs		
Suppressor	Active in blood	Very active	
Lymphocyte transformation			
with PHA	Poor	Poor	Normal
with *M. leprae*		Very poor	Normal
Delayed allograft rejection		4 days longer	2 days longer
Macrophage function	Deficient	Defective Unable to kill intracellular *M. leprae*	
Serum immunoglobulins	Raised	Normal	
Antibodies against			
M. leprae		Normal	Normal
Typhoid vaccine	Normal	Normal	Normal
Rheumatoid factor	May be +	±	Normal
Immune complexes	Yes	Yes	No
HLA	B8-A1	? DW3	
Erythema nodosum	Common	Occurs with treatment	Unusual
Amyloid	No	Yes with chronic ENL	No
Effect of steroids on immune response	Improves	Impairs	Impairs
Effect of transfer factor	? Improves	Improves	Unknown
OKT4:T8 ratio (see Table 13–1)	High at sites of activity Low in blood	Low	High

stomach, and uterus, and also particularly if they are treated by radiotherapy or chemotherapy. It is possible that treatment produces a granulomagenic substance that spreads to draining lymph nodes. A recent report draws attention to two patients with testicular carcinoma treated by radiotherapy or cytotoxic therapy who developed bilateral hilar lymphadenopathy containing sarcoid granulomas.[6] In most instances these isolated granulomatous tissue reactions are not true examples of multisystem sarcoidosis. With strict diagnostic criteria of sarcoidosis, most reported examples are local granulomas and, as such, are quite distinct from sarcoidosis.

The second facet is the diagnostic confusion between sarcoidosis and Hodgkin's disease, since multisystem granulomas are also commonly observed in the latter.[7] The difficulty usually arises in the interpretation of small specimens of aspiration liver biopsies or the occasional patient in whom the spleen is replaced by sarcoid tissue–obliterating tumour tissue. Intrathoracic Hodgkin's disease most frequently affects the upper mediastinum rather than hilar lymph nodes, and it is predominantly unilateral. In Hodgkin's disease the hilar nodes tend to fuse with the right cardiac border, whereas in sarcoidosis they stand away from the cardiac border. Both disorders show depression of cell-mediated immunity. In Hodgkin's disease, the Kveim-Siltzbach test is negative and serum angiotensin-converting enzyme levels are only raised in about 10 per cent of patients, compared with 60 per cent in sarcoidosis.

The final aspect is whether the impaired cellular immunity and anergy of sarcoidosis predispose to malignancy, as in patients with congenital immunodeficiency or those receiving immunosuppressant therapy.[8, 9] We have not observed an increased incidence of malignancy in 1,000 patients

Table 15–5. The Significance of a Granulomatous Reaction May Depend On the Age of the Patient

Age (years)	Description	Due to	Further Tests
0–5	Fundus oculi suggestive of retinoblastoma	*Toxocara choroiditis*	Check for eosinophilia, anaemia, lung infiltration
0–10	Cervical lymphadenitis draining sinus in the neck	Cat-scratch disease	Cat-scratch skin test and complement-fixation test for psittacosis group
0–15	Ulceration of limbs	Swimming pool granuloma	Isolate *Mycobaterium balnei*
20–40	Check all systems for multisystem sarcoidosis		
40–50	Obstructive jaundice	Primary biliary cirrhosis	Serum mitochondrial antibodies
		Cholelithiasis ⎫ Metastases ⎭	Ultrasound
Over 50	Sarcoid lymph nodes	Draining carcinomas, especially in patients receiving treatment	Think of cancer; more likely than sarcoidosis

Table 15–6. The Significance of a Granulomatous Reaction May Depend on the Environment of the Patient

Region	Disorder	Due to	Skin Test	Serum Antibody Test	Other Tests
Asia	Leishmaniasis	*Leishmania*		Formol gel	Giemsa-stained lymph node aspirate
Brazil, Egypt	Bilharziasis	*Schistosoma*	Yes		Find ova embedded in granuloma
Burma	Melioidosis	*Pseudomonas pseudomallei*	Yes	Yes	Culture organism
California	Coccidioidomyosis	*Coccidioides immitis*	Yes	Yes	Culture in Sabouraud's medium
India	Tuberculosis	*Mycobacterium tuberculosis*	Yes		Isolate organism, Chest radiography
Africa	Leprosy	*Mycobacterium leprae*	Yes		Scrapings
Ohio	Histoplasmosis	*Histoplasma capsulatum*	Yes	Yes	Culture in Sabouraud's medium

with sarcoidosis under personal supervision in London, and this has also been the Danish experience.[10] Further ongoing epidemiological studies in other populations around the world must be done.

MISCELLANEOUS GRANULOMAS

Among miscellaneous causes of sarcoid granulomas, the majority are local tissue reactions. The clinician must know of these to avoid labelling, a reaction to ruptured sebaceous cysts, for example, as a case of sarcoidosis. Similarly, a focal macrophage/sarcoid granulomatous reaction in lymph nodes following irradiation or chemotherapy is not sarcoidosis.

Granulomatous Mastitis[11, 12]

Granulomatous mastitis is a good example of a local sarcoid reaction resulting from leakage of fat-rich duct secretions. The condition presents as a painful, often post-partum, lump in young women. There are well-marked epithelioid granulomas, often with sterile micro-abscesses centered on ducts (Fig. 15–2). The condition is thus distinguished from the very rare involvement of the breast in sarcoidosis in which non-necrotic granulomas are randomly distributed.

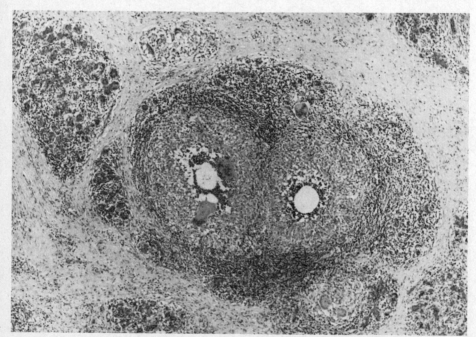

Figure 15–2. Granulomatous reaction with central necrosis within breast ducts. H & E × 128.

Foreign Body Granulomas

An interesting example is the not infrequent granulomatous response to a variety of woods, such as splinters or thorn pricks (Fig. 15–3). These may present as a localised nodule some considerable time after the local injury in the fingers. Recently it has been suggested that these lesions may be due to *Chlamydia* infections and are not merely foreign body reactions. A granulomatous reaction is also well recognised in pierced ears (Fig. 15–4) and following implantation of the spine of a sea urchin.[13]

Oil Granulomas

We have seen a number of examples of granulomatous responses to high-pressure grease gun injuries in motor mechanics (Fig. 15–5). Similar reactions may occur in response to paraffin, and we have also seen granulomas following injections in the treatment of haemorrhoids. We have also seen localised "paraffinomas" following cosmetic surgery to increase the size of the breast.

Sperm Granulomas

These may be seen within the body of the testis in granulomatous orchitis or in the epididymis. Similar reactions are also not uncommon following vasectomy (Fig. 15–6).

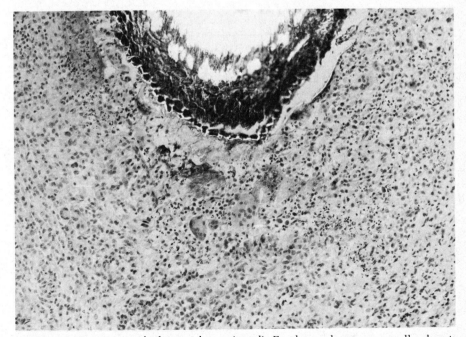

Figure 15–3. Foreign body granulomas (wood). Focal granulomas are usually absent, and the majority of giant cells are of a foreign body type. H & E × 65.

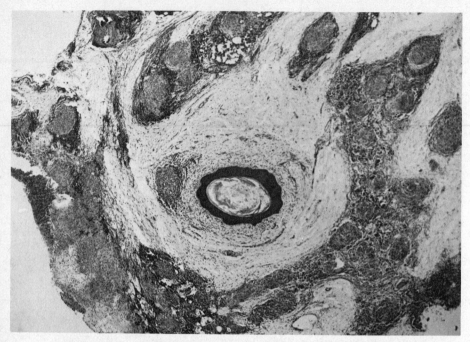

Figure 15–4. Earring granulomas around squamous-lined tract. H & E × 40.

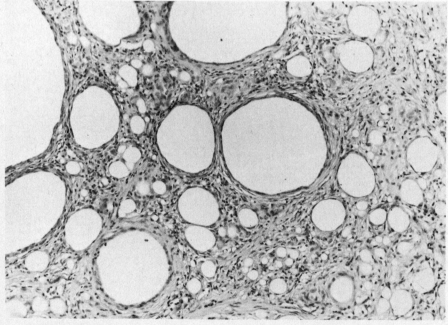

Figure 15–5. Grease gun (oleo) granuloma. Typical reaction to any injected oils. H & E × 80.

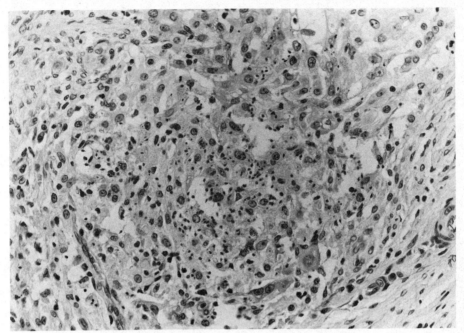

Figure 15–6. Sperm granuloma. Reaction to displaced lipids. Central sperm (black dots). H & E × 200.

IMMUNE COMPLEX DISEASES

These include conditions of unknown cause such as polyarteritis nodosa and giant cell arteritis that may produce a sarcoid-like reaction within vessel walls resulting from breakdown of elastica (Fig. 15–7). Rheumatoid disease is another example in which local skin nodules show palisading epithelioid and giant cells surrounding a central area of fibrinoid necrosis (Fig. 15–8).

TATTOO GRANULOMAS

Sarcoid granulomas may occur in areas of tattooing concomitant with or even preceding systemic sarcoidosis. Curiously they may be confined to only one colour, e.g., green.[14] Three patients with granulomas in light blue tattoos and simultaneous uveitis had no other evidence of systemic sarcoidosis.[15] Two of the three showed delayed skin reactivity to cobalt (considered to be the pigment in the tattoo), and excision of the involved area resulted in an improvement in the uveitis. It is likely that tattoo granulomas are examples of scar sarcoidosis (see Chapter 7).

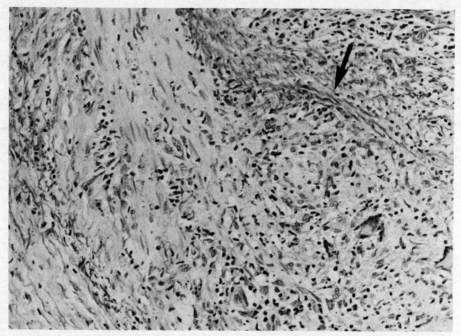

Figure 15–7. Giant cell arteritis. Response to fragmented elastica (arrow). H & E × 80.

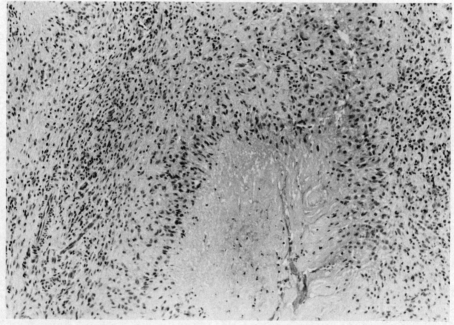

Figure 15–8. Rheumatoid nodule of skin. Extensive necrosis with palisade arrangement of surrounding epithelioid cells.

MALAKOPLAKIA[16]

This rare disease primarily but not exclusively affects the lower urinary tract and is associated with infection, usually by *Escherichia coli*. It is characterised by sheets of peculiar macrophages (von Hansenmann [vHC] cells) frequently containing targetoid calcified rounded bodies (Michaelis-Gutmann [MG] bodies) (Fig. 15–9), which bear a superficial resemblance to epithelioid cells and Schaumann's bodies. Focal granulomas and giant cells are not seen. vHCs are thought to arise from overloading of macrophages by incompletely digested organisms with accumulation of phagolysosomes, which transform into MG bodies. They are distinguishable by electron microscopy from epithelioid cells (see Chapter 3). Their rare occurrence outside the urinary tract, such as in the lungs, merits their inclusion in our differential diagnosis.

NECROTISING PROSTATIC GRANULOMAS[17]

Prostatic granulomas due to tuberculosis and as a reaction to displaced sperms are well recognised. A new entity has recently been described: necrotising granuloma following operative trauma. In six patients, necrotising (resembling rheumatoid nodules) granulomas and smaller foreign

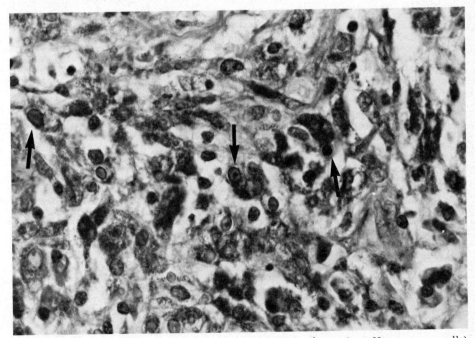

Figure 15–9. Malakoplakia showing numerous macrophages (van Hansenmann cells) overburdened with residual bodies forming Michaelis-Gutmann calcified bodies (arrows). H & E × 800.

body–type granulomas were found. Tuberculosis was excluded, and no foreign material was detected. The smaller hyalinised granulomas could easily be confused with those of sarcoidosis.

SUMMARY

All that glitters is not sarcoidosis. There are many unrelated causes of a sarcoid granuloma (Fig. 15–10).

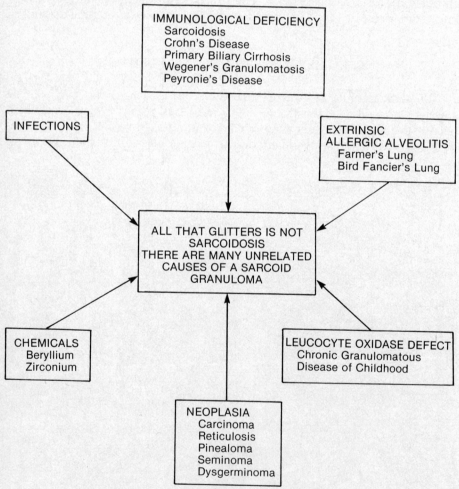

Figure 15–10. "All that glitters is not sarcoidosis."

REFERENCES

1. Luft BJ, Conley F, Remington JS. Outbreak of central nervous system toxoplasmosis in Western Europe and North America. Lancet. 1:781, 1983.
2. Warren KS. The pathology, pathobiology and pathogenesis of schistosomiasis. Nature. 273:609, 1978.
3. Ridley DS. Histological classification and the immunological spectrum of leprosy. Bull WHO. 51:451, 1974.
4. Narayanan RB, Bhutani LK, Sharma AK, Nath I. T cell subsets in leprosy lesions: in situ characterisation using monoclonal antibodies. Clin Exp Immunol. 51:421, 1983.
5. Ito Y, Toyama J, Morikawa S, Hirano T, Hirasawa K, Knoshita Y, Kanazawa Y. The production of granulomas in animals and men by a Proprionibacterium suspension and Yersinia. In Jones Williams W, Davies BH (eds): Sarcoidosis. Cardiff, Alpha and Omega Press. p 142, 1980.
6. Trump DL, Ettinger DS, Feldman MJ, Dragon LH. Sarcoidosis and sarcoid-like lesions—their occurrence after cytotoxic and radiation therapy of testis cancer. Arch Intern Med. 141:37, 1981.
7. Brincker H. Sarcoid reaction and sarcoidosis in Hodgkin's disease and other malignant lymphomata. Br J Cancer. 26:120, 1972.
8. Brincker H, Wilbek E. The incidence of malignant tumours in patients with respiratory sarcoidosis. Br J Cancer. 29:247, 1974.
9. Hoover R, Fraumeni JF. Risk of cancer in renal-transplant recipients. Lancet. 2:55, 1973.
10. Romer FK. Sarcoidosis and cancer—a critical review. In Jones Williams W, Davies BH (eds): Sarcoidosis. Cardiff, Alpha and Omega Press. p 567, 1980.
11. Fletcher A, Magrath IM, Riddell RH, Talbot IC. Granulomatous mastitis: a report of seven cases. J Clin Pathol. 35:941, 1982.
12. Davies JD, Burton TA. Postpartum lobular granulomatous mastitis. J Clin Pathol. 36:363, 1983.
13. Cooper P, Wakefield MC. A sarcoid reaction to injury by sea urchin spines. J Pathol. 112:33, 1974.
14. Farzan S. Sarcoid reaction in tattoos. NY Stat J Med. 77:1477, 1977.
15. Rorsman H, Delquist I, Jacobson S, Brehmer-Anderson E, Ehinger B, Linell F. Tattoo granulomas and uveitis. Lancet. ii:27, 1969.
16. McClure J. Malakoplakia. J Pathol. 140:275, 1983.
17. Lee G, Shepherd N. Necrotising granulomata in prostatic resection specimens—a sequel to previous operations. J Clin Pathol. 36:1067, 1983.

16

Aetiology

The cause of sarcoidosis remains unknown despite extensive research to uncover an infective agent, an immunological upset, an allergic mechanism, or a specific diathesis (Tables 16–1 and 16–2).

IS IT A KIND OF TUBERCULOSIS?

It was traditional to regard sarcoidosis as an odd form of tuberculosis, and the two diseases have certainly been confused with each other throughout this century (see pages 6, 202, and 238). This confusion continues because of the superficially similar epithelioid cell granulomas. But whereas those in sarcoidosis have minimal necrosis, tuberculous granulomas fuse and surround a lake of caseous necrosis. Sarcoidosis may be confused with tuberculosis, but there are crucial differences (see Table 15–3). *Mycobacterium tuberculosis* and other opportunistic mycobacteria are only rarely cultured from sarcoid tissue; these repeated failures have produced ingenious suggestions such as the mycobacteriophage theory.[1] Mycobacteriophage is common to both diseases, but mycobacteriophage antibodies are absent in sarcoidosis. The persistence of the phage without antibody explains why *M. tuberculosis* is not found in sarcoid tissue, giving rise to granulomatous sarcoidosis rather than tuberculosis. Research with animals[2] and humans[3]

Table 16–1. Comparison of an Autoimmune Disorder and Sarcoidosis

Indicators of an Autoimmune Disorder	Does Sarcoidosis Fit?
No recognised cause	Yes
Circulating autoantibodies	
Specific	Yes*
Non-specific	Not more frequent than normal
Hypergammaglobulinaemia	Yes
Histology: plasma cell infilration	No
Impressive response to	
Corticosteroids	Yes
Azathioprine	No
Anti-lymphocyte globulin	?
Cyclosporin	?

*Data from Favez G, Leuenberger P. Le diagnostic serologique de la sarcoidose. Rev Fr Mal Resp. 3:1037, 1975.

Table 16–2. Factors Contributing to the Aetiology of Sarcoidosis

?Infection	Background
Mycobacteria	HLA-B8/A1
Human	Familial recessive
Atypical	American black
Leprae	South African black
Protoplast	Irish
Virus	West Indian
Slow virus	Fertile women
Fungi, helminths, protozoa	Hormones
Lymphoproliferative response to	**Allergy**
Prolonged antigenaemia	Pine pollen
T4:8 ratio altered	Peanut dust
B cell overactivity	Clay eating
Circulating immune complexes	Pine pitch chewing
	Beryllium
	Zirconium

has failed to confirm this theory. A search for circulating antibodies to *M. tuberculosis* and other mycobacteria has also been inconclusive.[4]

Attempts have been made to detect granulomagenic components of *M. tuberculosis* in sarcoid tissue. The presence of mycolic acid esters has aroused interest,[5] but they are also found in normal tissue. Based on experimental studies, other granulomagenic components such as muramyl dipeptide (MDP) have been considered,[6] but they tend to be poor, second-rate granulomas consisting of foamy cells and epithelioid-like cells confined to the injection site and are not multisystem.

The world is witnessing decisive epidemiological differences, for the decline of tuberculosis is being followed by an upsurge of sarcoidosis. This fact must be included in any theory that sarcoidosis is a form of tuberculosis.

IS IT DUE TO A VIRUS?

Tissue culture has failed to uncover any virus despite many claims. The authors[7] and others have found high titres of Epstein-Barr virus (EBV) serum antibodies, but this reflects B cell hyper-reactivity rather than a causal relationship.[8] Sarcoid tissue homogenates have produced granulomas at sites of injection in the footpads of mice, suggesting transmission of a virus from sarcoid material,[9, 10] but the significance of these observations was undermined by other work indicating that these granulomas could also be produced by control normal lymph nodes.[11, 12]

Claims for a causal virus are longstanding, and, at various times, mumps, influenza, parainfluenza, Newcastle agent, and measles virus particles have been randomly isolated.

ANY OTHER CAUSAL INFECTION?

Bacteria

Propionibacterium acnes and *Yersinia* spp. have occasionally been cultured from sarcoid lymph nodes and their serum antibodies noted in 50 per cent of patients with sarcoidosis.[13] However, these organisms are ubiquitous, and their presence seems coincidental rather than causal. Likewise, *Brucella* sp. gives rise to hepatic granulomas but does not cause sarcoidosis.

Fungi

Fungi cause multisystem granulomatous disorders similar to sarcoidosis, and the confusion is heightened when the fungus is not cultured or its presence is not suspected by the histologist.

Aspergillus and *Nocardia* spp. may be occasional secondary invaders of chronic fibrotic pulmonary sarcoidosis; telltale eosinophils and other polymorphonuclears point to their presence in sarcoid tissue.

Protozoa

Infections such as leishmaniasis can mimic sarcoidosis, but the affected lymphoid tissue shows diffuse macrophage infiltration containing the parasite and only rarely produces focal epithelioid cell granulomas.

Toxoplasmosis

This may also mimic sarcoidosis. Histologically the granulomas are rarely as well developed as in sarcoidosis and usually consist of a small, five- to six-cell collection of macrophages containing the parasite. Again, note that without special stains, the diagnostic cysts can be easily overlooked. In endemic areas and in immunosuppressed subjects, such organisms must always be excluded.

Metazoa

Metazoa, particularly *Schistosoma* sp. *(Bilharzia)*, may cause multisystem granulomatous disease. Experimental studies have demonstrated similar immunological disturbances in both schistosomiasis and sarcoidosis.[14] However, the granulomas in schistosomiasis are rarely as florid as those in sarcoidosis, frequently include eosinophils, and are clearly distinguished by finding the central egg. Care must be taken, as the reaction is due to soluble glycoprotein fractions, so that the egg may not always be apparent. As eosinophils are not a feature of sarcoidosis, their presence should alert the pathologist to possible parasitic disease.

Mycoplasma[15, 16]

Mycoplasma sp. is occasionally cultured from sarcoid tissue. It is unlikely that it is primarily responsible, as the clinical features of *Mycoplasma* infections bear little resemblance to those seen in the syndrome of sarcoidosis.

Tuberculoid Leprosy

Tuberculoid lepropsy may mimic sarcoidosis both clinically and histologically in specific sites. Lepra bacilli are very sparse in these tissues and often cannot be detected. The skin lesions, erythema nodosum, peripheral lymphadenopathy, and neural lesions together with the immunological aberrations all combine to provide some superficial confusion (see Table 15–16).

IS IT AN IMMUNOLOGICAL ABERRATION?

The frequent involvement of lymph nodes and spleen, the raised serum immunoglobulins, the T and B cell involvement, and the presence of circulating immune complexes all point to a lymphoproliferative disorder with an immunological upset. Could this be a background factor providing an infective agent or other antigenic insult with a salubrious soil?

IS IT DUE TO HYPERSENSITIVITY?

Allergy (see Chapter 18, page 238)

Inhalation of pine pollen and peanut dust, clay eating, and pine pitch chewing have all been incriminated as contributory regional factors in different areas.[17] Extrinsic allergic alveolitis and hypersensitivity pneumonitis due to many different organic antigens mimic pulmonary sarcoidosis but not extrathoracic sarcoidosis.

Chemical

Beryllium[18–20] and zirconium[21] are known to produce sarcoid granulomas in the sensitised individual, but other elements do not seem to have this effect. Exhaustive skin testing with metals and other inorganic elements in sarcoidosis patients and controls has not revealed any peculiar hypersensitivity to chemicals. Skin tests for sarcoidosis, beryllium and zirconium disease, and leprosy are very similar in that a sarcoid granuloma is found at the injection site one month after inoculation. Each skin test is specific for its own disorder, and there is no overlap (see Table 13–2).

Sarcoid tissue is produced by a variety of agents including bacteria, fungi, viruses, helminths, chemicals, and even carcinoma. The common denominator of such dissimilar stimuli is unknown, but lipopolysaccharide has long been suspected. We have produced intradermal sarcoid granulomas in tuberculin-sensitive normal and sarcoidosis subjects using tuberculolipopolysaccharide.

IS IT AN AUTOIMMUNE DISORDER?

Indicators of an autoimmune process include iritis, sarcoid thyroiditis, erythema nodosum, and Sjögren's syndrome; hypergammaglobulinaemia; the occasional presence of odd non-specific circulating antibodies; and an impressive response to corticosteroids (see Table 16–1).

IS THERE A PREDISPOSITION?

Irish women in London and Puerto Ricans in New York are prone to erythema nodosum. Hormonal factors play some part, for erythema nodosum due to sarcoidosis is commoner in women during the child-bearing years and early pregnancy and also in women taking oral contraceptives. Sarcoid arthritis and erythema nodosum are most likely to occur in patients who are HLA-B8, A1, CW7, DR3. Patients with chronic (as compared with acute) sarcidosis are more likely to be HLA-B13 (see Table 13–3).

The occasional occurrence of familial sarcoidosis suggests possible genetic influences. The evidence suggests a racial predisposition to familial sarcoidosis, with a recessive mode of inheritance for susceptibility (see Chapter 18).

REFERENCES

1. Mankiewicz E, Walbeck M Van. Mycobacteriophages: their role in tuberculosis and sarcoidosis. Arch Environ Health (Chicago). 5:122, 1962.
2. Bowman BU, Amos WT, Geer JC. Failure to produce experimental sarcoidosis in guinea pigs with *M. tuberculosis* and mycobacteriophage DS6A. Am Rev Resp Dis. 105:85, 1972.
3. Bowman BU, Daniel TM. Further evidence against the concept of decreased phage neutralising ability of serum of patients with sarcoidosis. Am Rev Resp Dis. 104:908, 1971.

4. Chapman JS, Speight M. Further studies of mycobacterial antibodies in the sera of sarcoidosis patients. Acta Med Scand. (Suppl)425:61, 1964.
5. Nethercott SE, Strawbridge WG. Identification of bacterial residues in sarcoid lesions. Lancet. 2:1132, 1956.
6. Tanaka A, Emori K, Nagao S. Macrophage activation and epithelioid granuloma formation by a synthetic bacterial cell wall constituent. In Jones Williams W, Davies BH (eds): Sarcoidosis. Cardiff, Alpha and Omega Press. p 153, 1980.
7. James DG, Walker AN, Hamlyn AN. Immunology of sarcoidosis. In Iwai K, Hosoda Y (eds): Proc 6th Internat Conf Sarcoidosis. Tokyo, University Press. p 169, 1974.
8. Hirshaut Y, Glade P, Viera LO, Ainbender E, Dvorak D, Siltzbach LE. Sarcoidosis, another disease associated with serological evidence for herpes-like virus infection. N Engl J Med. 283:502, 1970.
9. Mitchell DN, Rees RJW. A transmissible agent from sarcoid tissue. Lancet. ii:81, 1969.
10. Mitchell LN, Rees RJW. The nature and physical characteristics of transmissible agent from human sarcoid tissue. Ann NY Acad Sci. 278:233, 1976.
11. Belcher RW, Reid JC. Sarcoid granulomas in CBA/J mice, histological response after inoculation with sarcoid and non sarcoid tissue homogenate. Arch Pathol. 99:283, 1975.
12. Iwai K, Takahashi S. Transmissibility of sarcoid specific granulomas in the footpads of mice. Ann NY Acad Sci. 276:249, 1976.
13. Ito Y, Toyama J, Morikawa S, Hirano T, Hirasawa K, Khoshita Y, Kanazawa Y. The production of granulomas in animals and men by a Proprionibacterium suspension and Yersinia. In Jones Williams W, Davies BH (eds): Sarcoidosis. Cardiff, Alpha and Omega Press. p 142, 1980.
14. Boros DL. Schistosomiasis mansoni. A granulomatous disease of cell mediated immune aetiology. Ann NY Acad Sci. 278:36, 1976.
15. Homma H, Okano H, Mochizuki H. An attempt to isolate mycoplasms from patients with sarcoidosis. In Levinsky L, Macholda F (eds): Proc 5th Internat Conf Sarcoidosis. Prague, Universita Karlova. p 101, 1971.
16. Hannuksela M, Jannson E. Isolation of a mycoplasma from sarcoid tissue. In Iwai K, Hosoda Y (eds): Proc 6th Internat Conf Sarcoidosis. Toyko, University Press. p 4, 1974.
17. Cummings MM, Dunner E, Schmidt BH, Barnwell JB. Concepts of epidemiology of sarcoidosis. Postgrad Med J. 19:437, 1956.
18. Jones Williams W. Beryllium disease, pathology and diagnosis. J Soc Occup Med. 27:93, 1977.
19. Jones Williams W, Williams R. The value of beryllium lymphocyte transformation tests in chronic beryllium disease and in potentially exposed workers. Thorax. 38:41, 1983.
20. Jones Williams W. Sarcoidosis 1977. Beitr Pathol. 160:325, 1977.
21. Shelley WB, Hurley HJ. The allergic origin of zirconium deodorant granuloma. Br J Derm. 70:75, 1958.
22. Favez G, Levenberger P. Le diagnostic sérologique de la sarcoidose. Rev Fr Mal Resp. 3:1037, 1975.

17

Treatment

Treatment is given in an endeavour to cure sarcoidosis. What is meant by cure has undergone spectacular metamorphosis during the last century (Table 17–1). Originally sarcoidosis was a dermatological curiosity, and the chronic skin lesions, usually lupus pernio, were persistent. There were occasional transient eruptions but they were hardly noticed. The introduction of x-rays provided serial standards of comparison; it was now possible to determine whether there was resolution of hilar adenopathy and pulmonary infiltration. Lung function tests provided yet another set of quantitative standards for comparison. Hyperglobulinaemia, hypercalcaemia, and hypercalciuria provided biochemical readings of remission and eventual cure. In more recent times, the Kveim-Siltzbach skin test, tests of T and B cell function, and serum angiotensin-converting enzyme have added further precision to our definition of cure. Corticosteroids constitute a mainstay of treatment around the world. They are administered to about one-half of afflicted patients (Table 17–2).[1] There are also several helpful alternative regimens (Table 17–3). The indications for steroid therapy follow.

EYES

The inflamed iris is treated with local atropine eye drops to maintain a dilated pupil. Topical corticosteroids should always be administered for iridocyclitis in the form of eye drops applied frequently during the day, re-

Table 17–1. Criteria of Cure of Sarcoidosis During the Last Century

Year	Criterion of Cure
1878	Skin lesions disappear
1914	Abnormal chest radiographical changes resolve
1935	Raised serum proteins revert to normal
1941	Kveim test becomes negative
1958	Hypercalcaemia and hypercalciuria return to normal calcium metabolism
1960s	Negative tuberculin skin test becomes positive
	In vitro phytohaemagglutinin transformation no longer anergic
	Lung function studies improve
1970s	Raised SACE level falls to normal
	BAL fluid reverts to normal
1980s	OKT4:OKT8 ratio returns to normal

Table 17–2. The Frequency with Which Oral Steroids
Were Prescribed for Sarcoidosis*

	Total No. of Patients	Oral Corticosteroids No.	%
London	537	185	34
New York	311	103	33
Paris	350	224	69
Los Angeles	150	97	65
Tokyo	282	193	68
Reading	425	107	25
Lisbon	89	42	47
Edinburgh	502	220	44
Novi Sad	285	263	92
Naples	624	249	40
Geneva	121	55	45
Total	3,676	1,738	47

*In a series of 3,676 patients attending special sarcoidosis clinics in nine different countries. Data from James DG, Neville E, Siltzbach LE, Turiaf J, Battesh JP, Sharma OP, et al. A worldwide review of sarcoidosis. Ann. NY Acad Sci. 278:321, 1976.

Table 17–3. Therapeutic Regimens in Sarcoidosis

Drug	Remarks
Prednisolone	The first line of treatment and the consistently most successful.
Non-steroidal Anti-Inflammatory Indomethacin Oxyphenbutazone	Helpful in acute exudative disease, such as erythema nodosum, polyarthralgia, acute iritis.
Immunosuppressives Azathioprine Cyclophosphamide Chlorambucil	When given together with steroids it is possible to halve the dose of steroids so it is steroid-sparing. When used alone, azathioprine may correct T cell irregularity and cyclophosphamide and chlorambucil may suppress B cell overactivity.
Chloroquine	Helpful in chronic fibrotic sarcoidosis involving skin and lungs. It should be given in a dose of 250 mg on alternate days only and limited to a course of nine months.
Potassium Para-aminobenzoate	Helpful in softening fibrotic lesions when given for at least nine months.
Methotrexate	Very helpful in controlling chronic skin lesions when given in a dose of 5 mg once weekly for 12 weeks.
Calcium chelating agents Effervescent phosphate Sodium phytate NA celluose phosphate	Only second best to steroids. They chelate calcium and prevent its absorption.
Cyclosporin A	Prevents experimental epithelioid cell granulomas.

inforced with a corticosteroid eye ointment at night. If there is no substantial and continuing improvement after one week, then the concentration of corticosteroid in the anterior segment of the eye may be increased with a local subconjunctival depot of cortisone. Oral prednisolone is indicated if local treatment does not lead to a rapid response or if ophthalmoscopy reveals posterior uveitis. The latter is best visualised by fluorescein angiography, which demonstrates leakage of dye due to retinal vasculitis. This responds well to oral prednisolone (40 mg daily). Treatment is continued for about three months, depending on the degree of involvement of other systems.

A raised intra-ocular pressure with local steroid eye drops is a signal to switch to fluorometholone eye drops, which are least likely to cause a rise in pressure, and also to consider Timoptol eye drops, which will return the intra-ocular pressure to normal.

INTRATHORACIC

Bilateral hilar lymphadenopathy is likely to subside without treatment, particularly if there is associated erythema nodosum. It has, therefore, been traditional worldwide not to treat Stage 1 hilar adenopathy. However, we now know from lung biopsy experience that there are active sarcoid granulomas in the lungs even when they are not evident in the chest radiograph. Raised serum angiotensin-converting enzyme (SACE) levels and radio-active gallium scans disclose their activity. The fire must surely be extinguished in these widespread granulomas, for otherwise they may lead eventually to pulmonary fibrosis. Therefore, we now treat hilar adenopathy if there is a significantly elevated SACE level (Fig. 17–1).

Pulmonary infiltration that remains static or worsens during the course of three months is an indication for oral prednisolone, again in an effort to prevent eventual irreversible pulmonary fibrosis (Fig. 17–2). Several factors influence the likelihood of resolution of the chest radiograph. The younger the patient, the more likely it is to clear. The presence of chronic skin lesions or bone cysts or both would confer an unfavourable prognosis, for these are the hallmarks of chronicity (see Fig. 4–4). Their presence would suggest that the pulmonary lesions are unlikely to subside. Substantial improvement in the chest radiograph is also related to the length of time prior to treatment. Results are considerably better in those treated within two years of onset of the disease.

Breathlessness. If this symptom is present, the patient has already reached a stage of irreversible pulmonary fibrosis or disturbed gas transfer. Oral steroids provide symptomatic relief but do not influence the natural history of the disease or its grave prognosis at the irreversible stage of breathlessness.

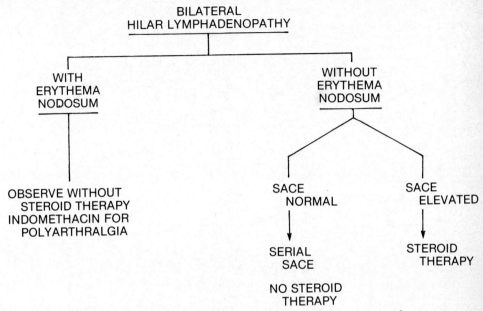

Figure 17–1. Treatment schedule for bilateral hilar lymphadenopathy.

Having proclaimed the value of steroid therapy in treating pulmonary sarcoidosis, it is as well to note the impact of steroids in our series in London (Table 17–4). Of the 700 patients with a chest x-ray abnormality, complete radiological resolution was eventually achieved in 362 patients (52 per cent); one-third achieved radiological resolution with steroids and two-thirds without steroids. Although there was no evidence that steroid therapy influenced the resolution of chest x-ray changes in pulmonary sarcoidosis, it is possible that without such treatment the number of patients with chronic persistent disease and its attendant morbidity might have been greater. Moreover, steroid therapy certainly provided symptomatic relief and overcame many manifestations of extrathoracic sarcoidosis.

Upper respiratory tract sarcoidosis may involve the pharynx and larynx with oedema, hoarseness, and stridor due to laryngeal obstruction. Intravenous steroids may be a matter of urgency, relieving life-threatening stridor. If given early enough, intravenous therapy may be sufficient to avoid tracheostomy.

SKIN

Steroid therapy is indicated for unsightly skin lesions such as lupus pernio involving the nose, lips, eyelids, cheek, and/or ears. Steroids shrink

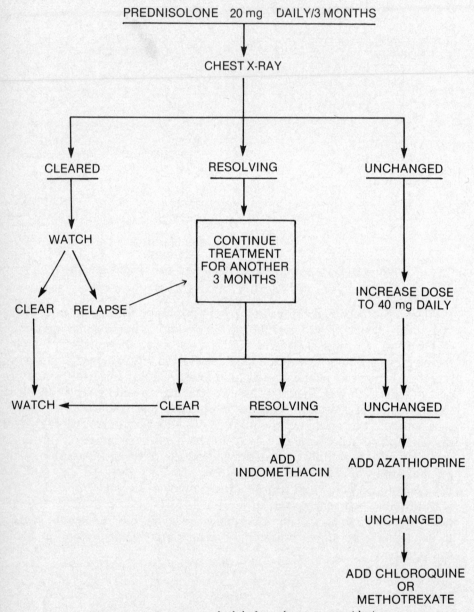

Figure 17–2. Treatment schedule for pulmonary sarcoidosis.

Table 17–4. Resolution of Intrathoracic Sarcoidosis in Relation
to Steroid Therapy

Chest X-ray Stage*	No. Patients	With Steroids			Without Steroids			Total Resolution	
		Total No.	Resolution No.	%	Total No.	Resolution No.	%	No.	%
1	458	208	93	45	250	175	70	268	59
2	150	82	28	34	68	31	46	59	39
3	92	56	10	18	36	25	69	35	38
Total	700	346	131	38	354	231	65	362	52

*Chest x-ray stage 1: Hilar lymphadenopathy only.
              2: Hilar adenopathy + pulmonary infiltration.
              3: Pulmonary infiltration without hilar adenopathy, ± fibrosis, scarring,
                 cavitation.

the disfiguring lesions, but they recur when treatment is discontinued.
Methotrexate, in a small dose of 5 mg once weekly, is also most effective in
overcoming unsightly lupus pernio (Fig. 17–3). When given with steroids, it
allows the dose of prednisolone to be reduced to a minimum (Table 17–5).

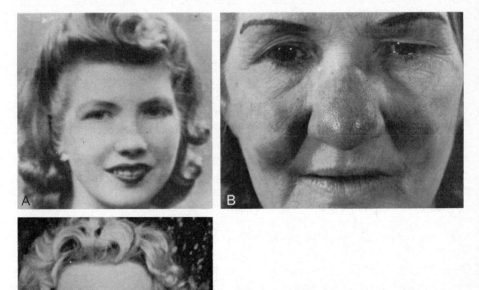

Figure 17–3. Lupus pernio. A, Before the
disease developed. B, The hideous deformity. C,
The disease treated and camouflaged.

Table 17–5. The Response of Lupus Pernio to Various Drugs

Treatment	Dose	Duration (mo)	Results
Prednisolone	Smallest possible	Shortest possible	Good
Chloroquine	250 mg on alternate days	9	Moderate
Methotrexate	5 mg weekly	3	Very effective
Potassium para-aminobenzoate	12 gm daily	12	Slight
Levamisole	150 mg daily	1	Unchanged
Antituberculous	Full	6	Unchanged

ABNORMAL CALCIUM METABOLISM

Disordered calcium metabolism is due to overactivity of calcitriol. The natural form, cholecalciferol (vitamin D_3), is metabolised first in the liver to 25-hydroxycholecalciferol, and then a second hydroxy group is added in the kidney to produce the potent, highly active 1,25-dihydroxycholecalciferol (calcitriol). Calcitriol causes increased intestinal calcium absorption, leading to hypercalcaemia and hypercalciuria. This can also be induced by sunlight. It is overcome swiftly by steroid therapy.

NERVOUS SYSTEM

The more acute the disease, the more likely it is to respond to systemic corticosteroids, which should be administered as soon as the diagnosis has been established. Resolution of neurosarcoidosis is more likely to occur in younger patients whose sarcoidosis has an explosive sudden onset. The response to treatment is better in those with accompanying erythema nodosum rather than chronic skin lesions; with acute rather than chronic uveitis; and with hilar adenopathy rather than old diffuse pulmonary infiltration.

Glandular involvement is common, particularly if there is disordered function; for example, dry eyes due to lacrimal gland involvement, dry mouth due to salivary gland enlargement, and hypersplenism due to sarcoidosis of the spleen. The indication for treatment is disordered function rather than anatomical enlargement of the gland in question.

HEART

It is easy to include involvement of the heart in a theoretical list of indications for corticosteroid therapy but much more difficult in practice to recognise myocardial sarcoidosis. It is, of course, suspected and treated when a patient with multisystem sarcoidosis develops cardiac arrhythmia or bundle branch block.

Treatment demands prolonged steroid therapy for resolution of the granulomas, chloroquine as an antifibrotic agent, beta blockers, nifedipine as a calcium antagonist, amiodarone or an equivalent as an anti-arrhythmic agent, and earlier use of pacemakers.

BONE

Bone cysts cause pain, swelling, and deformity of the hands and feet. Steroids provide relief of symptoms, but bone cysts persist despite treatment and symptoms recur when steroids are discontinued. Methotrexate and indomethacin are helpful alternative treatments.

OTHER DRUGS

Treatment may be necessary when there are contra-indications to steroid therapy.

Indomethacin

The activated macrophage produces interleukin-1, which, in turn, influences T4 helper lymphocytes. The macrophage–T lymphocyte feedback axis is prostaglandin-mediated. Indomethacin is a potent inhibitor of prostaglandin synthetase, and this may be its site and mode of action (see Fig. 13–3). It should be considered in acute exudative sarcoidosis. It is particularly valuable in patients with acute uveitis, phlyctenular conjunctivitis, sarcoid polyarthritis, and erythema nodosum.

Oxyphenbutazone

In a blind controlled trial comparing oxyphenbutazone, prednisolone, and a placebo in the management of pulmonary sarcoidosis, both active drugs were significantly better than the placebo.[2] Prednisolone and oxyphenbutazone were equally effective. Whereas one in six patients showed spontaneous regression of pulmonary sarcoidosis in six months, this trial showed that the number is increased by oxyphenbutazone or prednisolone to one in two patients. Not only does oxyphenbutazone influence the radiological picture but, like corticosteroids, it can prevent the development of sarcoid tissue, for it may prevent the evolution of sarcoid tissue in the Kveim-Siltzbach nodule. If oxyphenbutazone is to be successful it probably needs to be given within one year of the diagnosis of sarcoidosis in a dose of 100 mg four times daily for six months.

Chloroquine

The way in which chloroquine acts is unknown, but it controls some instances of chronic fibrotic sarcoidosis involving lungs and skin.[3] It is particularly helpful in the management of lupus pernio and pulmonary fibrosis. In view of its ocular toxicity, it should only be given in a dose of 200 mg on alternate days for up to nine months.

Methotrexate

This drug is helpful in the treatment of chronic skin lesions, particularly lupus pernio. Since it is known to cause hepatic fibrosis when taken daily for prolonged periods, we restrict it to a small dose of 5 mg taken once weekly for courses of three months. Patients are soon aware of its value, for it shrinks the cosmetically unacceptable lupus pernio effectively. However, when the course of treatment is discontinued, lupus pernio slowly recurs during the following three months. Repeated courses every six months, possibly in conjunction with oral steroids or chloroquine, and cosmetic camouflage represent the best treatment regimen at present.

Potassium Para-aminobenzoate (Potaba)

It is known to have an antifibrotic effect in Peyronie's disease, scleroderma, and rheumatoid arthritis. It is worth considering in pulmonary fibrosis and lupus pernio due to sarcoidosis. Three-gram envules should be taken by mouth four times daily for several months. This form of treatment is an alternative to corticosteroids, methotrexate, and chloroquine, and giving all four in rotation helps to overcome the undesirable long-term complications of any one drug.

Azathioprine (Imuran)[4, 5]

We have observed clinical improvement in 4, chest clearing in 2, and improved respiratory function in 1 out of a group of 10 patients given azathioprine. These 10 patients had already failed to respond to corticosteroids, oxyphenbutazone, and chloroquine, so they can be regarded as having hard-core chronic fibrotic sarcoidosis that has resisted all other therapy. Azathioprine may be helpful in sharing the burden of steroid therapy when the patient develops complications to steroids.

Radiotherapy

Before steroids were available, hilar adenopathy was treated by radiotherapy with good results. Corticosteroids swept aside this vogue, which is once again returning to favour. Williams and colleagues reported a patient with sarcoid meningitis associated with grand mal seizures.[6] The patient failed to respond to corticosteroid therapy but demonstrated improvement of symptoms, CT scan, and cerebrospinal fluid levels after receiving low-dose whole brain irradiation.

Cyclosporin A

Cyclosporin A is a fungal metabolite with interesting immunosuppressant properties. It seems to act selectively on immunocompetent T lymphocytes and has virtually no effect on other white blood cells. It acts at an early stage of T cell stimulation, interfering with interleukin-2 production (see Fig. 13–3) and preventing organ rejection, hence its current popularity in the field of organ transplantation. Cyclosporin A exerts profound effects on experimental epithelioid cell granulomas produced in rats by subcutaneous injections of various opportunistic mycobacteria. In a daily oral dose of 20 mg/kg, it prevented the formation of epithelioid cell granulomas or the development of caseous necrosis in the course of one month. Macrophages containing well-preserved mycobacteria accumulated at the local site and in the regional lymph node, but there was no generalisation of infection. Inhibition of T lymphocyte activation by cyclosporin A prevented harmful mycobacterial infection in this experimental model. The mycobacterial infection remained circumscribed and even showed signs of regression. Preliminary studies in acute sarcoidosis with a dose of 5 mg/kg body weight are being undertaken.

Sodium Cellulose Phosphate (Calcisorb*)

This is indicated for the treatment of absorptive hypercalciuria associated with recurrent formation of renal calculi. It is an ion-exchange compound with a particular affinity for divalent cations. It binds calcium ions in the lumen of the stomach and intestine; the calcium complex is excreted harmlessly in the faeces. It is a white-to-beige fibrous powder. Each 5-gm sachet binds 250 mg of calcium. The usual adult dose is 5 gm three times daily.

Effervescent Phosphate†

Each effervescent phosphate tablet provides 500 mg elemental phosphorus to bind calcium. The daily adult dose is 1 to 2 gm.

---

*Riker Laboratories.
†Sandoz.

INEFFECTIVE AND HARMFUL REGIMENS

Calciferol. This is positively harmful, for it gives rise to hypercalcaemia and hypercalciuria. Multivitamin preparations containing vitamin D are best avoided during pregnancy. Likewise, *ultraviolet light* should not be administered to patients with active sarcoidosis.

Antituberculous Chemotherapy. This therapy is of no benefit in sarcoidosis. The only possible indication is when the physician is undecided whether the patient has sarcoidosis or tuberculosis.

Invalidism. Patients with sarcoidosis should not become invalids in sanatoriums. They should be encouraged to return to work, to become pregnant, and to lead normal lives.

Levamisole. This anthelmintic has been extensively investigated for its immunotherapeutic potential in restoring impaired cellular immunity in cancer and auto-immune disorders. A short-term trial of 150 mg daily for four weeks in 22 patients with chronic sarcoidosis had no effect on the clinical course or the skin reactivity of patients with active chronic sarcoidosis.

REFERENCES

1. James DG, Neville E, Siltzbach LE, Turiaf J, Battesti JP, Sharma OP, et al. A worldwide review of sarcoidosis. Ann NY Acad Sci. 278:321, 1976.
2. James DG, Carstairs LS, Trowell JS, Sharma OP. Treatment of sarcoidosis: Report of a controlled therapeutic trial. Lancet 2:526, 1967.
3. Siltzbach LE, Teirstein AS. Chloroquine therapy in 43 patients with intrathoracic and cutaneous sarcoidosis. Acta Med Scand. (Suppl)425:302, 1964.
4. Sharma OP, Hughes DTD, James DG, Naish P. Immunosuppressive therapy with azathioprine in sarcoidosis. *In* Levinsky L, Macholda F (eds): Transactions 5th Internat Conf Sarcoidosis. Prague, Universita Karlova. p 635, 1971.
5. Israel HL. Effects of chlorambucil and methotrexate in sarcoidosis. *In* Levinsky L, Macholda F (eds): Transactions 5th Internat Conf Sarcoidosis. Prague, Universita Karlova. p 632, 1971.
6. Grizzanti JN, Knapp AB, Schecter AJ, Williams MH. Treatment of sarcoid meningitis with radiotherapy. A J Med. 73:605, 1982.

18

Epidemiology

WORLDWIDE DISTRIBUTION

Sarcoidosis has a worldwide distribution, but it is more frequently recognised in sophisticated communities. Whenever tuberculosis or leprosy is rampant, sarcoidosis is in eclipse, but as tuberculosis and leprosy are brought under control, sarcoidosis becomes more evident. Thus, worldwide epidemiological surveys should seek sarcoidosis in the wake of declining tuberculosis and leprosy. In Uruguay, the eradication of tuberculosis and the widespread use of miniature radiography brought to light a surprising frequency of sarcoidosis[1] (Table 18–1). Data on 3,676 patients in 11 cities—London, New York, Paris, Los Angeles, Tokyo, Reading, Lisbon, Edinburgh, Novi Sad, Naples, and Geneva—revealed that the prevalence of the disorder is surprisingly similar in various parts of the world.[2]

BLACK POPULATIONS

United States

Much shoe leather has been expended on the epidemiology of sarcoidosis in the US. It is evident that sarcoidosis is about 10 times more frequent in the American black population than in the American Caucasian population. Interestingly, the sarcoidosis profile is also different in the two groups.[3] One-third of the black sarcoidosis patients compared with only 2 per cent of the Caucasian sarcoidosis patients were born in the Southeastern United States. Female preponderance was only noted in the black patients. Respiratory symptoms, pulmonary infiltration, fever, weight loss, and skin and eye lesions are significantly more common in blacks than in Caucasians. Serum globulin elevations are more frequent, and eosinophilia is largely confined to black patients.

South Africa

The previously held view that sarcoidosis is rare in the black population of South Africa is no longer tenable. A survey at Groote Schuur Hospital,

233

Table 18–1. Prevalence of Pulmonary Sarcoidosis per 100,000 of Population Examined*

Area		Prevalence
New York	Blacks	80
	Puerto Ricans	30
Sweden		55–64
Uruguay		60
Denmark		53
Germany		41
Hungary		40
Eire		40
West Berlin		30
United Kingdom		27
Cape Town	Blacks	27
	Coloureds	17
	Caucasians	6
Norway		26
New Zealand		6–24
Czechoslovakia		23
Holland		21
London		19
Switzerland		16
Leipzig		13
Japan		12
Italy		11
Yugoslavia		11
Poland		10
Northern Ireland		10
France		10
Canada		10
Finland		9.2
Australia		9
Scotland		8
Argentina		1–5
Spain		3
Israel		1.6
Korea		1
Brazil		0.2
Portugal		0.2
Rumania		120 (total)
Taiwan		6 (total)

*A composite of figures reported at various International Sarcoidosis Conferences.

Cape Town, reveals a prevalence rate per 100,000 of 17 in coloured, 27 in black, and 6 in Caucasian patients. Deforming arthritis and widespread and florid skin lesions were found only in black patients. This accounts for the mistaken diagnosis of leprosy in the past. Morrison reported a series of 18 black patients with sarcoidosis;[5] all suffered from gross skin lesions, including lupus pernio, papules, nodules and plaques (some psoriasiform), a few lesions in the sites of old injury, and nail dystrophies. Two-thirds of the afflicted patients had intrathoracic involvement, one-half had bone cysts, and one-third had ocular involvement. What is of particular interest in this survey is that some of these patients had been mistakenly incarcerated in a leprosy institution. The diagnosis of sarcoidosis was only entertained when patients had failed to improve on antileprotic, antituberculous, and anti-syphilitic treatment. This reminds one of the bad old days when patients with sarcoidosis were also mistakenly detained in tuberculosis sanatoriums. In those days sarcoidosis was considered when patients failed to respond to antituberculous chemotherapy or when the tuberculin skin test was found to be negative.

Western Europe

Sarcoidosis is also frequent in the Caucasian population of Scandinavia and throughout Europe. It is most frequent in sophisticated diagnostic centres. In our London series of 818 patients, the place of birth was the United Kingdom in 74 per cent of patients, the West Indies in 10 per cent, and Ireland in 8 per cent.

A mass chest radiographical survey carried out in London revealed that intrathoracic sarcoidosis was particularly prevalent in West Indians and also in the Irish (Table 18–2).[6–10] The prevalence rate per 100,000 of those born in Britain is 27, rising to 97 in Irish men, 213 in Irish women, 197 in West Indian men, and 170 in West Indian women, all living in North London (see Table 18–2). What are the figures for the Irish staying home in Ireland? During the years 1970 through 1973, the Irish Mass Radiography Board did 1,000,000 examinations and found a rate of 40 per 100,000, the same rate as that of the English at home and considerably less than that of Irish immi-grants.[10] One explanation is that the Irish x-rayed at home were in the 15- to 29-year age group compared with the 20- to 40-year age group of the Irish migrants. Or could it be that the Irish and West Indians become exposed to some factor in London to which the indigenous population has become relatively immune?

Just as London sees much sarcoidosis among its migrants from the British West Indies, so does Paris see it in its migrants from Martinique. Is this due to genetic predisposition or to environmental factors confronting susceptible individuals migrating from a rural to an urban community? Is

Table 18–2. Prevalence of intrathoracic Sarcoidosis Among Ethnic Groups in London*

| | Rate Per 100,000 | |
Birthplace	Male	Female
United Kingdom	27	27
Ireland	97	213
British Caribbean	197	170

*Data from Brett Z. Prevalence of intrathoracic sarcoidosis among ethnic groups in London. *In* Levinsky L, Macholda F (eds): Proc 5th Internat Conf Sarcoidosis. Praha, Universita Karlova. p 238, 1971.

the breeding ground for sarcoidosis in their native environment or within the sophisticated new world to which they adapt themselves? It may be a bit of both.

Eastern Europe

Djuric and colleagues studied the features of sarcoidosis in Novi Sad and Belgrade (Yugoslavia), Debrecen (Hungary), Istanbul (Turkey), Hamburg (West Germany), and Warsaw (Poland) along precisely the same lines as the worldwide survey, so it is possible to compare their findings with those of the rest of the world[11] (Table 18–3). The profile of sarcoidosis in Eastern Europe is similar to that in other parts of the world. Levinsky and colleagues have noted a fivefold increase in Löfgren's syndrome in Czechoslovakia, particularly in women, largely because of its better recognition by doctors.

Japan

The statistics for sarcoidosis in Japan underline the adage that you will find it if you look hard enough. A Japan Sarcoidosis Committee carried out six sarcoidosis surveys across the nation from 1960 to 1978.[12] These surveys detected 5,038 cases with a rate of 3 per 100,000 population. A sixth survey was completed in 1978, revealing a fourfold increase of the prevalence rate to 12 per 100,000 population. The determination, pertinacity, and efficiency of this committee will undoubtedly increase these rates still further in the future.

Based on their studies in various parts of Japan, the committee members feel that sarcoidosis is induced by an infective agent, is prevalent in cool climates and influenced by seasonal ecological variations, and develops in predisposed individuals.

Sarcoidosis is extremely rare in the rest of Asia, possibly because of the considerable amount of tuberculosis still present.

India

Sarcoidosis was rare in India, presumably because widespread tuberculosis and leprosy obscured it. Until 1981, only 75 patients with systemic sarcoidosis had been reported in India[13]; since that survey it is being increasingly recognised and will undoubtedly become commonplace by the end of this decade. Patterns of presentation, tissue involvement, and results of investigation are surprisingly similar to those noted in other parts of the world (Table 18–4).

Table 18–3. Comparisons of Sarcoidosis Around the World

Features	Western Worldwide	Eastern Europe
Total number	3,676 (100%)	2,066 (100%)
Women	57	57
Black	10	0.3
Age under 40 years at presentation	68	70
Onset		
Routine chest x-ray	40	64
Chest x-ray Stage 0	8	4
1	51 (65)†	58 (65)
2	29 (49)	30.5 (31)
3	12 (20)	7.5 (3)
Total % resolution	(54)	(55)
Intrathoracic involvement	87	96
Lymph nodes	22	8
Erythema nodosum	17	11
Eyes	15	4
Other skin	9	5
Spleen	6	1
Parotid	4	1.5
Nervous system	4	1
Bone cysts	3	3.5
Positive Kveim-Siltzbach test	78	73
Negative tuberculin test	64	58
Hyperglobulinaemia	44	44
Hypercalcaemia	11	12
Treated with steroids	47	59.5
Mortality due to		
Sarcoidosis	2.2	1
Other causes	1.4	1

*Percentages given for ease of comparison.
†Percentage resolution of chest x-ray changes at each stage in parentheses.

Table 18–4. Percentage Comparison of Sarcoidosis in India Compared with Worldwide Series and Eastern Europe

Feature	India	Worldwide	Eastern Europe
Female	41	57	57
Intrathoracic involvement	98	87	96
Skin lesions	20	26	16
Ocular involvement	10	15	4
Parotid enlargement	7	4	1.5
Nervous system	10	4	1
Positive Kveim test	89	78	73
Negative tuberculin skin test	71	64	58
Hypercalcaemia	47	11	12
Hyperglobulinaemia	44	44	44

SOCIAL FACTORS

Sarcoidosis is confined to human beings. Nothing quite like it has so far been found in the veterinary world, and this may be one reason why nobody has yet succeeded in transmitting it to an experimental animal. Non-specific local sarcoid tissue reactions are, of course, easily produced in animals, but these are quite different from the generalised multisystem disease sarcoidosis. Is man uniquely susceptible because of his peculiar social habits, or are certain humans particularly vulnerable as a consequence of their internal or external environment? We collected data in an endeavour to detect any predisposing factor[8] (Tables 18–5 and 18–6).

EXPOSURE TO TUBERCULOSIS

The relationship between sarcoidosis and tuberculosis has been hotly debated. The evidence for and against tuberculosis as an aetiological factor in sarcoidosis has been admirably summarised by Siltzbach,[14] who concludes that one disease is not a cause of the other. In our series, exposure to the tubercle bacillus was the same (27 per cent) in both sarcoidosis and control subjects; tuberculosis did not seem to give rise to or to protect against sarcoidosis. Similar results were obtained in a study of 74 patients, predominantly coloured, in Georgia.[15, 16] A study in Denmark compared the geographical distribution of sarcoidosis with the tuberculin pattern in the general population (as represented by participants in a mass immunisation campaign), the geographical tuberculin pattern in cattle, and the geographical pattern for the incidence of pulmonary tuberculosis. There was no correlation between sarcoidosis and these factors.[17] Likewise, there was no association between sarcoidosis and tuberculosis in an Oklahoma study.[18]

FAMILY DISEASE PATTERNS

A family history of other chest diseases including carcinoma of the bronchus, chronic bronchitis, and congestive cardiac failure was sought from our patients. There was no significant difference in the incidence of these illnesses in patients and control subjects.

INHALANTS

The distribution of sarcoidosis was found to be similar to that of pine trees, i.e., both predominate in the Southeastern United States.[18-20] In Britain, 2 per cent of control patients and 3 per cent of sarcoidosis subjects expressed exposure to conifers. Our findings served to minimise the association

Table 18–5. Questionnaire Answered by 327 Sarcoidosis Patients and 127 Control Subjects

---

Name
Mr. Mrs. Miss
Single, Married,
  Widowed

Date of birth
Place of birth

No.
Year of onset
Diagnosis (controls)

---

1. Occupation: Type of work
    Do you come in contact with:
    (a) Hay
    (b) Farm animals (specify types)
    (c) Trees or sawdust (specify types)
    (d) Dusts of coal, silica, asbestos, beryllium; other dusts (specify types).

---

2. Hobbies
   Material used

---

3. Places of residence in this country and abroad (residence of over 6 months only need be
    included from the age of 16 to the present)
Town   Country   Dates

---

4. Were any of the places you lived in close to woods or forests?
Place   How Close   Kind of trees

---

5. Pets: Have you ever kept pets in the family or been in contact with them?
Types of pets   Approximate dates

---

6. List fuels used for home heating or cooking and indicate approximate dates of use.

---

7. At what age did you start smoking   stop smoking
    Do you smoke manufactured cigarettes (Tipped/untipped)   yes/no
                                         Cigars   yes/no
                                         Hand-rolled cigarettes   yes/no
                                         Pipe   yes/no

---

8. Obstetric: Number of pregnancies
             Year   Outcome (full term, abortion, etc.)
    Pica (during pregnancy or at any other time)   Details of feeding
    Menstrual history

---

9. Further family history: Age if   Date of   Age at   Cause of
                                             alive   death   death   death

   Mother
   Father
   Brothers and sisters
   Children
   Details of any family history suggestive of:
     Sarcoidosis (skin, chest, eye disease)
     Tuberculosis
     Allergies

---

between sarcoidosis and pine trees and are in line with similar epidemiological data from Denmark, Japan, Switzerland, Belgium, and Uruguay. Exposure to mineral dusts or vegetable or animal sources is not a significant factor in London. The possible significance of clay eating as an aetiological factor in sarcoidosis was investigated in Georgia, where it was observed that this habit occurred twice as often in a group of sarcoidosis patients as in the controls.[16] Although the clay contains a small amount of beryllium, which is

Table 18–6. History of Contact in 327 Sarcoidosis Patients Compared with 127 Controls

Contact	Sarcoidosis No.	%	Other Diseases No.	%
Known contact with tuberculosis	87	27	33	27
History of chest disease in relatives	48	15	39	31
Possible respiratory irritants				
Pine	8	3	3	3
Other trees	55	19	19	16
Cotton	7	2	0	0
Clay	1	1	0	0
Minerals	59	20	17	24
Domestic fuel				
Coal	241	79	99	77
Gas	192	63	90	70
Oil	70	23	30	23
Electricity	125	41	55	43
Pets				
Dogs	181	55	64	52
Cats	143	43	59	47
Birds	73	22	29	23
Smoking materials				
Cigarettes	121	37	43	34
Pipes	27	9	1	1
Cigars	17	5	2	2
Pregnancies (no. of children per woman)	1.4		1.6	
Breast-fed children	141/260	54	68/125	54
Urban birthplace	210	63	87	65
Rural birthplace	117	37	40	34
Urban domicile for more than 10 years	282	86	114	90
Rural domicile for more than 10 years	104	32	31	24

known to provide sarcoid granulomata, clay eating was not regarded as a primary aetiological factor but rather as a secondary, or trigger, mechanism. In our series in sarcoidosis and control patients, there was no difference in the degree of exposure to clay or to dusts from coal, other minerals, or cotton. Nor was there any difference in the type of household fuel used or in the contact with domestic pets or allergens produced by them.

TOBACCO AND ALCOHOL

In our London series tobacco and alcohol consumption patterns were similar in both sarcoidosis and control subjects.

PREGNANCY

Pregnancy might be a predisposing factor, since the number of children borne by sarcoidosis patients (3.1 children per woman) was greater than that of controls (2.4 children per woman), although male sarcoidosis patients had the same sized families as controls.[16] We found no differences in family size, pregnancies, or breast-feeding patterns in sarcoidosis and control subjects.

ICEBERG SYNDROME

Sarcoidosis is an iceberg syndrome, for many forms of the disease lie undetected (Fig. 18–1). We must dig deeper to uncover latent forms of the disease. As new techniques emerge, they help to detect excitingly new clinical manifestations of the disease. When fluorescein angiography was introduced, it revealed leaking retinal veins, which were promptly sealed by corticosteroid therapy. Likewise, brain scans brought a new dimension, visualising space-occupying sarcoid granulomas and hydrocephalus. It is to be hoped that radioactive scans will uncover latent myocardial sarcoidosis.

EPIDEMIOLOGICAL SEARCH

Following are recommendations for a concentrated search for sarcoidosis and its possible causes in nature:

1. In setting up a sarcoidosis clinic, three disciplines should combine to make it a joint clinic comprising chest physician, dermatologist, and ophthalmologist. The increased yield would be fruitful.

2. Mass chest x-ray surveys should be conducted in the wake of tuberculosis and leprosy. Those responsible for the eradication of these

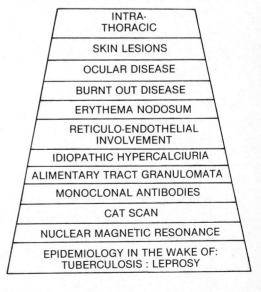

Figure 18–1. Sarcoidosis is an iceberg syndrome.

INTRA-THORACIC

SKIN LESIONS

OCULAR DISEASE

BURNT OUT DISEASE

ERYTHEMA NODOSUM

RETICULO-ENDOTHELIAL INVOLVEMENT

IDIOPATHIC HYPERCALCIURIA

ALIMENTARY TRACT GRANULOMATA

MONOCLONAL ANTIBODIES

CAT SCAN

NUCLEAR MAGNETIC RESONANCE

EPIDEMIOLOGY IN THE WAKE OF: TUBERCULOSIS : LEPROSY

Table 18–7. Familial Occurrence of Sarcoidosis*

Authors	Year	Relationship	Location
Martenstein[21]	1923	2 sisters	Germany
Sellbei and Berger[22]	1926	3 sisters and 2 brothers	Vienna
Dressler[23]	1938	2 brothers	Switzerland
	1939	Brother and sister	
MacCormac[24]	1940	2 sisters	London
Richter and Richter[25]	1941	2 sisters	Germany
van Buchem[26]	1946	2 brothers	Tilburg
Robinson and Hahn[27]	1947	2 brothers; 4 brothers	Baltimore
Bickerstaff[28]	1949	2 brothers	Ireland
Sherer and Kelly[29]	1949	Identical twins	US
Klingmuller[30]	1951	Mother and son; 2 sisters	Germany
Gilg[31]	1952	Identical twins	Copenhagen
Rogers and Netherton[32]	1954	Identical twins	Cleveland
Van Zwanenberg and Barry[33]	1955	3 brothers and 1 sister	England
Swirsky and Lowman[34]	1955	Brother and sister	Connecticut
Moriarty[35]	1956	2 sisters	England
Warin[36]	1958	Mother and son; brother and sister	England
Kendig, Peacock, and Ryburns[37]	1959	3 sisters	Virginia
Baer[38]	1960	2 brothers and 2 sisters	Texas
Kinoshita, Ogima, and Aoki[39]	1966	Mother and 2 daughters	Japan
Beresford[40]	1970	Mother and daughter; mother and son	England
Sharma, Johnson, and Balchum[41]	1971	3 brothers and 1 sister	Los Angeles
Wiman[42]	1973	4 families (21 members, 3 generations)	Sweden
Ito, Ogima, and Kinoshita[43]	1973	12 families (25 members)	Japan
James et al.[44]	1974	5 families (11 members)	London
Sharma et al.[45]	1978	16 families (33 members)	London and Los Angeles
Kendig[46]	1976	1 family (4 children)	Virginia
Israel and Washbourne[47]	1980	8 patients (7 black)	Philadelphia
Hosoda et al.[48]	1980	16 siblings (9 parent-child; 2 husband-wife)	Japan

*Data from references 21 through 48.

Table 18–8. Features of 31 Patients with Familial Sarcoidosis Compared with Sarcoidosis Overall

Feature	Sarcoidosis Overall No.	%	Familial Sarcoidosis No.	%
Women	500	61	21	70
Black	79	10	17	55
Age at presentation				
Under 40 years	604	74	22	71
Over 40 years	214	26	9	29
Total	818	100	31	100
Tissues				
Lungs	716	88	31	100
Erythema nodosum	251	31	3	10
Lymph nodes	225	27	8	26
Eyes	224	27	7	22
Skin (other than EN)	147	21	5	16
Spleen	101	12	2	6
Parotid	52	6	3	10
Bone cysts	31	3	3	10
Nervous system	77	9	1	3
Intrathoracic				
Stage 0	118	14	0	42
1	458	65	13	32
2	150	22	10	26
3	92	13	8	
Tests				
Tuberculin skin test negative	488/782	70	20/26	76
Kveim-Siltzbach skin test positive	430/658	65	11/20	55
Corticosteroid therapy necessary	344	42	19/31	61
Mortality due to				
Sarcoidosis	25	3	1	3
Other causes	23	3	2	6

disorders should send follow-up teams for the detection of sarcoidosis. It would be of particular interest to know its incidence in the Caribbean and South America.

3. In addition to chest x-rays, other markers of granulomatous inflammation, including serum angiotensin-converting enzyme and serum lysozyme levels, should be sought.

4. Skin test surveys using tuberculin and Kveim-Siltzbach antigen should be conducted.

FAMILIAL SARCOIDOSIS

During this century, familial sarcoidosis has been reported in 160 or so patients in the world literature[21–48] (Table 18–7). We have reported 16 families in whom 33 persons had sarcoidosis[45] (Table 18–8). It is more frequent in monozygotic rather than dizygotic twins. The modes of presentation, multisystem involvement, course, and prognosis are similar in familial and sporadic sarcoidosis. The commonest family relationship is a brother and sister with sarcoidosis, followed by a mother-offspring relationship. We have not observed it in a father-offspring relationship, which is exceedingly rare. Wiman noted it once,[42] and Scharkoff has observed this rare pairing in East Germany.[49] Sarcoidosis in both husband and wife is not unique. Most sarcoidologists with large series have seen such an example. It is too rare to point to an infective background, but it would suggest a common environmental basis. The evidence in our familial series indicates a recessive mode of inheritance.[44]

The British Thoracic and Tuberculosis Association collected data on 59 families in Britain in whom there was more than one case of sarcoidosis.[50] The most striking finding was the significant preponderance of like-sex over unlike-sex pairs among both siblings and parent-child associations. Their observed preponderance of monozygotic (four) over dizygotic (one) twin pairs concordant for sarcoidosis is strongly suggestive of a genetic predisposition.

There has been a recent interesting study of familial sarcoidosis in the Irish Republic, where sarcoidosis has a prevalence rate of 33 per 100,000 individuals screened. The study group comprised 85 patients with biopsy-proven sarcoidosis with a sibling pool of 416 individuals. Eleven siblings derived from nine families were identified as having sarcoidosis, providing a high prevalence of 10 per cent with familial sarcoidosis.[51]

REFERENCES

1. Purriel P, Naverrete E. Epidemiology of sarcoidosis in Uruguay and other countries of Latin America. Am Rev Resp Dis. 84:155, 1961.
2. James DG, Neville E, Siltzbach LE, Turiaf J, Battesti JP, Sharma OP, Hosoda Y, Mikami R, Odaka M, Villar TG, Djuric B, Douglas A, Middleton W, Karlish AJ, Blasi A, Olivieri D, Press P. A worldwide review of sarcoidosis. Ann NY Acad Sci. 278:321, 1976.
3. Israel HL, Wishburne JD. Characteristics of sarcoidosis in black and white patients. In Jones Williams W, Davies BH (eds): Sarcoidosis. Cardiff, Alpha and Omega Press. p 497, 1980.
4. Benatar S. Sarcoidosis in South Africa. In Jones Williams W, Davies BH (eds): Sarcoidosis. Cardiff, Alpha and Omega Press. p 508, 1980.
5. Morrison JGL. Sarcoidosis in the Bantu. Br J Dermatol. 90:649, 1974.
6. Anderson R, Brett GZ, James DG, Siltzbach LE. The prevalence of intrathoracic sarcoidosis. Med Thorac. 20:152, 1963.
7. James DG, Brett GZ. Prevalence of intrathoracic sarcoidosis in Britain. Acta Med Scand. (Suppl)425:115, 1964.
8. Hall G, Sharma OP, Naish P, Doe W, James DG. The epidemiology of sarcoidosis. Postgrad Med J. 45:241, 1969.
9. Brett Z. Prevalence of intrathoracic sarcoidosis among ethnic groups in London. In Levinsky L, Macholda F (eds): Proc 5th Internat Conf Sarcoidosis. Praha, Universita Karlova. p 238, 1971.
10. Comminsky J. Sarcoidosis among the Irish. Lancet. 1:366, 1976.

11. Djuric B, Handi L, Vezendi S, Celikoglu S, Breyne H, Jaroszewicz W, Krychniak W, Piotrowski M, Zych D, Jevric S, Draganic B. Sarcoidosis in six European cities. *In* Jones Williams W, Davies BH (eds): Sarcoidosis. Cardiff, Alpha and Omega Press. p 527, 1980.
12. Hosoda Y, Iwai K, Odaka M. Recent epidemiological features of sarcoidosis in Japan. *In* Jones Williams W, Davies BH (eds): Sarcoidosis. Cardiff, Alpha and Omega Press. p 519, 1980.
13. Gupta SM, Chatterjee S, Roy M. Clinical Profile of Sarcoidosis in India. Lung India. 1:1, 1982.
14. Siltzbach LE. Sarcoidosis and mycobacteria. Am Rev Resp Dis. 97:1, 1968.
15. Comstock GW. Tuberculosis studies in Muscogee County, Georgia. I. Community-wide tuberculosis research. Publ Hlth Rep. 64:259, 1949.
16. Comstock GW, Keltz H, Sencer DJ. Clay eating and sarcoidosis. A controlled study in the State of Georgia. Am Rev Resp Dis. 84:130, 1961.
17. Horwitz O. Geographic epidemiology of sarcoidosis in Denmark: 1954–1957. Am Rev Resp Dis. 84:135, 1961.
18. Shook B, Hammersten J, Levinson R, Goldsmith JB, Cummings MM. Trans US Veterans' Administration 21st Res Conf Pul Dis. p 186, 1962.
19. Cummings MM, Dunner E, Schmidt RH, Barnwell JB. Concepts of epidemiology of sarcoidosis. Postgrad Med J. 19:437, 1956.
20. Cummings MM, Dunner E, Williams JH. Epidemiologic and clinical observations in sarcoidosis. Ann Intern Med. 50:879, 1959.
21. Martenstein H. Knochveranderungen bei lupus pernio. Z Haut (Ceschlechtskr). 7:308, 1923.
22. Sellbi J, Berger M. Sarkoide Gescjwulste in eine Familie. Arch Derm Syph (Wien). 150:47, 1925.
23. Dressler M. Boeck'sche Krankheit der Lungen bei Geschwisern. Schweiz Mschr Wschr. 19:417, 1938.
24. MacCormac H. Schaumann's disease in two sisters. Acta Med Scand. 103:152, 1940.
25. Richter P, Richter W. Beitrag zur Klinik der Besnier-Boeck-Schaumannscher Erkrankung. Derm Wschr. 113:797, 1941.
26. Van Buchem RSP. On morbid conditions of the liver and diagnosis of Besnier-Boeck-Schaumann disease. Acta Med Scand. 124:168, 1946.
27. Robinson RCV, Hahn RD. Sarcoidosis in siblings. Arch Intern Med. 80:249, 1947.
28. Bickerstaff ER. The familial aspects of sarcoidosis. Br J Tuberc. 43:112, 1949.
29. Sherer JP, Kelly RT. Sarcoidosis in identical twins. N Engl J Med. 240:328, 1949.
30. Klingmuller G. Der Morbus Boeck in der Familie. Derm Wschr. 124:119, 1951.
31. Gilg I. Boeck's sarcoid in identical twins. Acta Dermatovener. (Suppl)29:108, 1952.
32. Rogers FJ, Netherton EW. Sarcoidosis in identical twins. JAMA. 155:974, 1954.
33. van Zwanenberg D, Barry M. A case of sarcoidosis and 3 cases of atypical tuberculosis in one family. Lancet 1:483, 1955.
34. Swirsky MY, Lowman RM. Sarcoidosis in siblings. N Engl J Med. 252:476, 1955.
35. Moriarty MA. Sarcoidosis in siblings. J Irish Med Assoc. 38:7, 1956.
36. Warin RR. Familial sarcoidosis. Br J Dermatol. 70:250, 1958.
37. Kendig EL, Peacock RL, Ryburns S. Sarcoidosis: Report of three cases in siblings under 15 years of age. N Engl J Med. 260:952, 1959.
38. Baer RB. Familial sarcoidosis: epidemiological aspects with notes on a possible relationship to the chewing of pine pitch. Arch Intern Med. 105:60, 1960.
39. Kinoshita Y, Ogima I, Aoki S. Three cases of sarcoidosis occurring in two generations of a family. Jap J Clin Med. 23:190, 1966.
40. Beresford OD. Familial sarcoidosis. Jap J Chest Dis. 30:297, 1971.
41. Sharma OP, Johnson CS, Balchum OJ. Familial sarcoidosis: report of four siblings with acute sarcoidosis. Am Rev Resp Dis. 104:255, 1971.
42. Wiman LG. Familial occurrence of sarcoidosis. *In* Iwai K, Hosoda Y (eds): Proc 6th Internat Conf Sarcoidosis. Tokyo, Tokyo University Press. p 22, 1973.
43. Ito Y, Ogima I, Kinoshita Y. Familial sarcoidosis in Japan. *In* Iwai K, Hosoda Y (eds): Proc 6th Internat Conf Sarcoidosis. Tokyo, Tokyo University Press. p 30, 1974.
44. James DG, Piyasena KHG, Neville E, Walker AN, Hamlym AN. Possible genetic influences in familial sarcoidosis. Postgrad Med J. 50:664, 1974.

45. Sharma OP, Neville E, Walker AN, James DG. Familial sarcoidosis: a possible genetic influence. Ann NY Acad Sci. 278:386, 1976.
46. Kendig EL. Familial sarcoidosis. Ann NY Acad Sci. 278:400, 1976.
47. Israel HL, Washbourne JD. Characteristics of sarcoidosis in black and white patients. Analysis of 162 recent cases. *In* Jones Williams W, Davies BH (eds): Sarcoidosis. Cardiff, Alpha and Omega Press. p 497, 1980.
48. Hosoda Y, Iwai K, Odaka M, Hiraga Y, Ito, T, Furniye T, Mikami R, Yaragawa H, Hashimoto T, Shigematou I, Chiba Y. Recent epidemiological features of sarcoidosis in Japan. *In* Jones Williams W, Davies BH (eds): Sarcoidosis. Cardiff, Alpha and Omega Press. p 519, 1980.
49. Scharkoff T. Personal communication, 1978.
50. British Thoracic and Tuberculosis Association. Familial association in sarcoidosis. Tubercle. 54:87, 1973.
51. Brennan NJ, Crean PA, Long D, Fitzgerald M. Familial sarcoidosis in an Irish population. Thorax. 37:228, 1982.

INDEX

Note: Page numbers in *italic* type indicate illustrations; page numbers followed by *t* refer to tables.

Aetiology, of sarcoidosis, 216–221
    epidemiological search, recommenda-
        tions for, 241–243
Age, in cardiac sarcoidosis, 114t
    in granulomatous reactions, significance of,
        205t
    in incidence of sarcoidosis, 38, 39t, 40t, 41t
    in lupus pernio, 107t
    in osseous sarcoidosis, 135t, 136
Alimentary tract, 144–155. See also specific
        organs.
    granulomas of, 145t
    management of, 149t
Alkaline phosphatase, 170, 171t
Allergy, as cause of sarcoidosis, 219
Alveolitis, extrinsic allergic (EAA), differen-
        tial diagnosis of, 62–63
    source of dust antigens in, 65t
    vs. sarcoidosis, distinguishing features
        of, 65t
    in pulmonary sarcoidosis, 55
Anergy, 174
    helper to suppressor cell ratios in, 174, 175t
Angiotensin-converting enzyme (ACE), as
        marker of sarcoid activity, 193t
    monitoring of, 54–55
    serum (SACE), 168–170
        correlating tests with, 194, 194t
        levels of, in disease states, 168t
        in sarcoidosis, 168t, 171t
Antibody, antimitochondrial, in liver granu-
        lomas, 185t
    antinuclear, in liver granulomas, 185t
    smooth muscle, in liver granulomas, 185t
Antituberculous chemotherapy, dangers of,
        232

Arteritis, giant cell, sarcoid-like reaction in,
        211, *212*
Aspergillosis, clinical features of, 201t
Asteroid bodies, in giant cells, 25, *26*
Auto-antibodies, in liver granulomas, 185t
Autoimmune disorders, vs. sarcoidosis, 216t
Autoimmunity, 184, 185t
    as cause of sarcoidosis, 220
Azathioprine (Imuran), in treatment of sar-
        coidosis, 230

B lymphocytes, activity of, 177–178
Bacteria, as cause of sarcoidosis, 218
Beryllium, as cause of sarcoidosis, 219
    lymphadenopathy and, 128
Beryllium disease, vs. sarcoidosis, 60–62, 62t
Beryllium skin test, 180, 181t
Besnier, 5
Bibliography, on sarcoidosis, sources of, 10
Bilharziasis, geographical regions of, 206
    tests for, 206t
Bilirubin, serum, 170
Biochemistry, of sarcoidosis, 163–173
Blacks, incidence of sarcoidosis in, 233–235
    in South Africa, 233–235
    in United States, 233
Blastomycosis, clinical features of, 201t
Boeck, Caesar, 2t, 3
    historic patient of, *xi*, 6, 7
    Carl W., 3
    Christian, 3
Bone, 134–135
    sarcoidosis of, age and sex in, 135t, 136
    clinical features of, 135t

Bone (*Continued*)
  sarcoidosis of, healing in, 141–142
    lytic lesions in, 136, *138, 139,* 141
    multiple fractures in, *139*
    race in, 135t, 136
    radiology in, 136–141
    symptoms of, 136
    treatment of, 229
Bone cyst(s), in osseous sarcoidosis, *138,* 141
Bone lesions, destructive, 136
  in sarcoidosis, frequency of, 135t
    healing of, 141-142
    lytic, 136, *138, 139,* 141
    permeative, 136
Brain, lesions of, in neurosarcoidosis, 91, *92,*
  93
Breathlessness, in sarcoidosis, treatment of,
  224
Bronchial wall stenosis, in pulmonary sarcoi-
  dosis, *56,* 58
Broncho-alveolar lavage (BAL), 54–55, 178
  sarcoidosis vs. idiopathic pulmonary fibro-
  sis in, 55t
Bronchocentric granulomatosis, differential
  diagnosis of, 61t, 67
Bronchoscopy, in histological diagnosis, 31
Bronchostenosis, *56,* 58
Brucella, granulomas due to, 204
Brucellosis, lymph node granulomas in, 122
  management outline for, 149t

Calciferol, harmful effects of, 232
Calcisorb (sodium cellulose phosphate), in
  treatment of hypercalciuria, 231
Calcitriol, abnormal, in sarcoidosis, 165
Calcium, levels of, abnormal, in sarcoidosis,
  163–166, 164t, 165t, 171t
  metabolism of, abnormal, in sarcoidosis,
  166
    treatment of, 228
Cardiac sarcoidosis, 112–117. See also *Heart,*
  sarcoidosis of.
Cat scratch disease, lymphadenopathy in,
  123, *123*
Cell markers, in evaluation of sarcoidosis,
  196, 196t
Cheilitis, granulomatous (Melkersson-Rosenthal syndrome), *xii,* 151–152, *151*
Chemicals, as cause of sarcoidosis, 219
Childhood, polyarthropathy in, differential
  diagnosis of, 159–160
  sarcoidosis of, 155–160
    chest involvement in, 158
    clinical features of, 158t
    extrathoracic lesions in, 158–159, 158t
    prognosis in, 159
    race and sex in, 156, 158t
    symptoms of, 156, 158t

Chloroquine, in treatment of sarcoidosis, 230
Churg-Strauss syndrome, differential diagnosis of, 61t, 67
Circulating immune complexes (CIC),
  178–179
Cirrhosis, primary biliary, histological appearance of, *148*
  lymph node granulomas in, 128
  management outline for, 149t
  vs. sarcoidosis, 146, 147t
Clay eating, in aetiology of sarcoidosis, 239
Coccidioidomycosis, clinical features of, 201t
  geographical regions of, 206t
  tests for, 206t
Complement, levels of, 178
Conjunctiva, biopsy of, 33–34
  blind, 85–87
  involvement of, in sarcoidosis, 85–87, *86*
Conjunctival follicles, 85, *86*
Conjunctivitis, phlyctenular, 85
Corticosteroids, in treatment of sarcoidosis,
  222, 223t
Crohn's disease, lymph node granulomas in,
  128
  management outline for, 149t
  vs. sarcoidosis, clinical features of, 153t
Cryptococcosis, clinical features of, 201t
Cyclosporin A, in treatment of sarcoidosis,
  231
Cystic pneumatosis, lymph node granulomas
  in, 128

Dactylitis, sarcoid, *140,* 142
Death, sudden, in cardiac sarcoidosis,
  113–114
Diagnosis, differential, 199–215
  of pulmonary sarcoidosis, 59–68
  histological, 30–36
    tissue distribution patterns in, 30t

Earring granulomas, 209, *210*
Echocardiography, in cardiac sarcoidosis, 116
Electrocardiography, in cardiac sarcoidosis,
  114
Enterocolitis, *Yersinia,* 204
Environment, significance of, in granulomatous reactions, 206t
Epidemiology, of sarcoidosis, 233–246
  exposure to tuberculosis in, 238, 240t
  family patterns in, 238
  history of contacts in, 240t
  social factors in, 238, 239t
Epithelioid cell(s), 176–177
  histology of, *xi,* 6, *7,* 21–24, *22–24*
  types of, distribution of, *xi, 24*

Epithelioid cell granulomas, pulmonary interstitial, *56*
Erythema nodosum, 97–100
  appearance of, *99*
  arthralgia preceding, vs. acute rheumatism, 142t
  as feature of sarcoidosis, 43
  causes of, 100, 101t, *102*
    clinical features associated with, *102*
  conditions associated with, 101t
  duration of, 46
  early history of, 7–8
  geographical distribution of, *103*
  incidence of, 97t, 98t
  seasonal, *99*
Europe, Eastern, incidence of sarcoidosis in, 236, 237t
  Western, incidence of sarcoidosis in, 235, 237t
Examination, clinical, diagrammatic plan for, *41*
Eyes, involvement of, in sarcoidosis, 42. See also *Ocular sarcoidosis*; *Conjunctiva*, etc.
  treatment of, in sarcoidosis, 222–224

Familial sarcoidosis, 243–244
  incidence of, 242t
  vs. sarcoidosis overall, comparative features of, 243t
Farmer's lung, sarcoid granulomas and alveolitis in, *64*
Fibrosis, idiopathic pulmonary, vs. sarcoidosis, 55t
  in sarcoid granulomas, 26–27, *27–29*
Fingers, deformities of, in osseous sarcoidosis, 136, *137, 140,* 142
Francisella tularensis, lymphadenopathy associated with, 123
Fungal diseases, granulomatous, mimicking sarcoidosis, 201t
Fungi, as cause of sarcoidosis, 218
  infective granulomas due to, 199, 200t

Galactorrhoea-amenorrhoea syndrome, 93
Gallium scanning, in evaluation of sarcoid activity, 195–196, *195*
Gastrointestinal system, 144–145. See also specific organs.
Genetics, in aetiology of sarcoidosis, 220, 244
Giant cell arteritis, sarcoid-like reaction in, 211, *212*
Giant cells, histological appearance of, *xi, 6, 7*
Granuloma(s), collagen replacement in, *28, 29*
  foreign body, 209, *209*
  formation of, secondary "antigen" in, *29*

Granuloma(s) (*Continued*)
  hepatic, 146
    febrile, management outline for, 149t
  infective, agents of, 199–205, 200t
    differential diagnosis of, 199–205
  Kveim, distribution of cell types in, 186t
  lymph node, cellular features of, 121t
    disorders associated with, 119t
  necrotising prostatic, 213–214
  of alimentary tract, 145t
    localised, 154
    management of, 149t
  oil, 209
  reticulin replacement in, *27*
  sarcoid. See also *Sarcoid granuloma(s)*.
    distribution of cell types in, 186t
    formation of, 184–186, *184, 185*
      factors contributing to, *184*
    pathogenesis of, 184–186, *184, 185*
  sperm, 209, *211*
  tattoo, 211
Granulomatosis, bronchocentric, differential diagnosis of, 61t, 67
Granulomatous disease, age of patient in, significance of, 205t
  classification of, 17–20, 19t
  environment in, significance of, 206t
  of childhood, chronic, lymphadenopathy in, 125
Granulomatous lung disease, chemical, differential diagnosis of, 60–62, 62t
  differential diagnosis of, 60–68, 61t
Granulomatous mastitis, in differential diagnosis, 208, *208*

Hamazaki-Wesenburg bodies, 25
Heart, sarcoidosis of, 112–117
  age and sex in, 114t
  cardiac biopsy in, 34, 116
  clinical features of, 43, 114t
  clinical presentations in, 112–113
  diagnostic tests for, 114–116
  fibrosis of bundle of His in, *115*
  myocardial granulomas in, *115*
  prognosis in, 116–117
  sites of cardiac granulomas in, *113*
  treatment of, 116–117, 228–229
Heerfordt's syndrome, 87–88
  historical background of, 9
Histiocytosis-X, vs. sarcoidosis, differential diagnosis of, 63–64, 66t
  X bodies in macrophage of, *66*
Histocompatibility (HLA) antigens, 182–184
Histology, diagnostic, 30–36
  tissue distribution patterns in, 30t
Histoplasmosis, clinical features of, 201t
  geographical regions of, 206t
  lymphadenopathy in, 125, *125*
  tests for, 206t

History, of sarcoidosis, 1–16
first published account in, 1, 4
landmarks in, 2t
multisystem recognition in, 6–7
HLA antigens, 182–184
significance of, in sarcoidosis, 183t
Hodgkin's disease, hepatic granulomas in, 147
management outline for, 149t
vs. sarcoidosis, comparative features of, 127t
differential diagnosis of, 205
Hutchinson, Jonathan, 1–3
Hydrocephalus, in neurosarcoidosis, 92
Hydroxyprolinuria, 171, 171t
Hypercalcaemia, in sarcoidosis, 163, 164t, 171t
as index of sarcoid activity, 193, 193t
Hypercalciuria, in sarcoidosis, 163, 164t, 165t, 171t
as index of sarcoid activity, 193, 193t
Hyperglobulinaemia, 164t, 166–168, 171t
Hyperprolactinaemia, 93
Hypersensitivity, as cause of sarcoidosis, 219
Hypersensitivity pneumonitis. See Alveolitis, extrinsic allergic.
Hypertension, portal, sarcoid, 145–146
pulmonary, in cardiac sarcoidosis, 113
Hyperuricaemia, 170, 171t
Hypogammaglobulinaemia, lymphadenopathy and, 128
Hypothalamus, in cerebral sarcoidosis, 93–94

Iceberg syndrome, sarcoidosis as, 241, 241
Immune complex diseases, in differential diagnosis, 211
Immune complexes, circulating (CIC), 178–179
Immune response serum suppressor factors, 179
Immunity, cellular, 174–176
humoral, 177–184
Immunoblastic (angioimmunoblastic) lymphadenopathy, 128
Immunoglobulins, serum, in sarcoidosis, 164t, 166–168, 171t
Immunological disorders, as cause of sarcoidosis, 219
lymph node granulomas and, 128
Immunology, 174–191
markers of sarcoid activity in, 194–195
of leprosy and sarcoidosis, 207t
Imuran (azathioprine), in treatment of sarcoidosis, 230
Inclusion bodies, of epithelioid and giant cells, 24–25, 25, 26
India, incidence of sarcoidosis in, 236, 237t
Indomethacin, in treatment of sarcoidosis, 229

Infection(s), as cause of sarcoidosis, 217t, 218–219
granulomatous, differential diagnosis of, 199–205
granulomatous lymph nodes in, 119–125, 119t
Inhalants, incidence of sarcoidosis and, 238–240
Intestine, 153–155
Intrathoracic sarcoidosis, 49–68
clinical features of, 41
differential diagnosis of, 59–68
radiological, 60t
incidence of, among London ethnic groups, 235t
in Western Europe, 235
stages of, 49–54
chest x-ray resolution, 52t
effect of steroid therapy on, 53t, 54
Stage 1 of, 53
Stage 2 of, 53
Stage 3 of, 53–54
treatment of, 224–225, 226
results of, 227t
Invalidism, harmful effects of, 232
Iridocyclitis, acute, vs. chronic, xii, 80, 80t, 82
Iritis, acute, xii, 80, 82
historical background of, 8

Japan, incidence of sarcoidosis in, 236
Joints, sarcoidosis of, 142

Keloid, sarcoid, 110. See also Scars.
Keratoconjunctivitis sicca, 85, 88
Kidney, sarcoidosis of, 160
clinical features of, 44
Kidney function tests, 170
Killer (K) cells, activity of, 177
Kveim granuloma, distribution of cell types in, 186t
Kveim-Siltzbach skin test, 34–36, 179–182
comparative results of, 35t
historical background of, 9–10
positive, sarcoid granulomas in, xii, 180

Lacrimal gland, involvement of, in sarcoidosis, 44
Laryngeal mucosa, sarcoidosis of, 69, 70t, 71, 72
histological appearance of, xi, 71
Leishmania, infective granulomas due to, 199, 200t
Leishmaniasis, geographical regions of, 206t
lymphadenopathy in, 124
tests for, 206t

Lepromin reaction, in leprosy, 180, 181t
Leprosy, and sarcoidosis, immunology of, 207t
  geographical regions of, 206t
  lepromatous, lymphadenopathy in, 122
  lepromin reaction in, 180, 181t
  tests for, 206t
  tuberculoid, and sarcoidosis, 219
    clinical appearance of, *204*
    vs. sarcoidosis of upper respiratory tract, 74t
Levamisole, ineffectiveness of, 232
Liver, 144–148
  granulomas of, auto-antibodies in, 185t
    causes of, 145t
    differential diagnosis of, 146–148
    management of, 148, 148t
  infections of, vs. sarcoidosis, 146
Liver biopsy, 31–32
Liver function tests, 170
Locomotor system, sarcoidosis of, 132–143
  clinical features of, 43–44
Löfgren's syndrome, 88
  historical background of, 8
Lung(s). See also *Pulmonary sarcoidosis.*
  farmer's, sarcoid granulomas and alveolitis in, *64*
  fibrosis of, in pulmonary sarcoidosis, *57*
  granulomatous diseases of, differential diagnosis of, 60–68, 61t
  pathology of, in pulmonary sarcoidosis, 55–58
Lung function tests, in evaluation of sarcoid activity, 192
Lupus pernio, 100–108
  age and sex in, 107t
  appearance of, *103*
  clinical features of, 43
  experimental model of, 108
  historical background of, 5
  of scalp, *xii, 104*
  plaques of, *105, 106,* 111
    histologic appearance of, *106*
  racial incidence of, 107t
  treatment of, 225
    results of, 108, 108t, *227,* 228t
  vs. sarcoidosis, clinical features of, 107t
Lymph node biopsy, 31
Lymph nodes, 118–119
  granulomas of, cellular features of, 121t
    disorders associated with, 119t
    immunological disorders and, 128
    in alimentary tract, 128–129
    mineral particles in, 127–128
    sarcoid, histological appearance of, *120*
Lymphadenitis, cholegranulomatous, lymph node granulomas in, 128
  dermatopathic, lymphadenopathy in, 129, *129*
Lymphadenopathy, bilateral hilar, 41

Lymphadenopathy (*Continued*)
  bilateral hilar, treatment of, 224, *225*
  drug-induced, 130
  hilar, duration of, *47*
    radiographic changes in, *50, 51*
  immunoblastic (angioimmunoblastic), 128
  lymphangiographic, 130
  sarcoid, 118, *120*
  silicone, 130, *130*
Lymphangiographic lymphadenopathy, 130
Lymphocytes, abnormal activity of, 174
Lymphokines, activity of, 188
  in epithelioid granulomas, 25–26
Lymphoma, malignant, sarcoidosis associated with, 127
Lymphomatoid granulomatosis, differential diagnosis of, 61t, 67
Lymphoreticular system, sarcoidosis of, 118–131
  clinical features of, 43
Lysozyme, serum, 171t

Macrophages, activated, 176
Macular sarcoidosis, *83*
Maculo-papular eruptions, 108–109, *109*
Malakoplakia, in differential diagnosis, 213, *213*
Mastitis, granulomatous, in differential diagnosis, 208, *208*
Melioidoisis, geographical regions of, 206t
  tests for, 206t
Melkersson-Rosenthal syndrome (granulomatous cheilitis), 151–152, *151*
Meningeal sarcoidosis, *92*
Meningitis, in neurosarcoidosis, 90, 90t
Metazoa, as cause of sarcoidosis, 218
  infective granulomas due to, 200–202, 200t
Methotrexate, in treatment of sarcoidosis, 230
Monokines, activity of, 188
Mortimer, Mrs., 5–6, *6*
  historic report on, 5
Mouth, 151–152
Muscle, 132–134
  sarcoid granuloma in, *133*
Muscle biopsy, 33
Muscle nodules, 133–134
  granulomatous, *134*
Mycobacteria, infections with, lymph node granulomas and, 119–122, 119t
  infective granulomas due to, 202–203
Mycobacterium balnei, swimming-pool granuloma due to, 203
Mycobacterium leprae, leprosy granulomas due to, 203
Mycobacterium tuberculosis, granulomas due to, 202
Mycoplasma, as cause of sarcoidosis, 219
Myopathy, chronic, 133

Nasal bone, sarcoidosis of, 69, 70t
Nasal mucosa, sarcoidosis of, 69, 70, 70t
Nasal septum, perforation of, 69
Neoplasia, in differential diagnosis, 205–208
lymph node granulomas in, 126, 126
Nervous system, involvement of, in sarcoidosis, 42. See also *Neurosarcoidosis.*
in upper respiratory tract sarcoidosis, 73
Neurosarcoidosis, 89–95
CAT scanning in, 95
chest radiography in, 95
changes in, 95t
clinical features of, 42, 90t
differential diagnosis of, histological, 94
posterior nerve root in, 93
prognosis in, 94
treatment of, 228
NK (natural killer) cells, activity of, 177

Ocular sarcoidosis, clinical features of, 42, 78
distribution of lesions in, 77–80, 79
historical background of, 8, 77
incidence of, 78t, 79
syndromes of, 87–89, 87
treatment of, 222–224
Oil granulomas, 209, 210
Osseous sarcoidosis. See *Bone, sarcoidosis of.*
Osteitis tuberculosa multiplex cystica, 7
Oxyphenbutazone, in treatment of sarcoidosis, 229

Palsy, facial, in neurosarcoidosis, 89, 90t, 91
Papilloedema, 84, 85
in neurosarcoidosis, 89, 90t
Parotid gland, in sarcoidosis, 148–149
clinical features of, 44, 151t
enlargement of, 150
histological appearance of, 150
Pathology, of sarcoidosis, 21–37
Peritoneoscopy, in histological diagnosis, 32
Pharyngeal mucosa, sarcoidosis of, 69, 70t
Phosphate, abnormal levels of, in sarcoidosis,
166
effervescent, for calcium binding, 231
Plaques, of lupus pernio, 105, 106, 111
Pneumatosis, cystic lymph node granulomas
in, 128
Pneumonitis, hypersensitivity. See *Alveolitis,
extrinsic allergic.*
Polymyositis, acute, 132
Polyneuropathy, in neurosarcoidosis, 91
Portal hypertension, sarcoid, 145–146
Positron tomography, in pulmonary sarcoi-
dosis, 59
Potassium para-aminobenzoate (Potaba), in
treatment of sarcoidosis, 230

Predisposition, in incidence of sarcoidosis,
220
Pregnancy, sarcoidosis in, 160
incidence of, 240–241
Prostatic granulomas, necrotising, 213–214
Proteins, serum, in sarcoidosis, 166–168
Protozoa, as cause of sarcoidosis, 218
infective granulomas due to, 199, 200t
Pseudomonas mallei, lymphadenopathy associated with, 123
Pulmonary hypertension, in cardiac sarcoidosis, 113
Pulmonary sarcoidosis, 41
course of, 47
differential diagnosis of, 59–68
pathology of, 55–58
physiology of, 58–59
radiographic changes in, 52
treatment of, 224–225, 226
worldwide distribution of, 234t
Pulmonary talc granulomatosis, vs. sarcoidosis, 62, 63
Purple lupus. See *Lupus pernio.*

Race, in childhood sarcoidosis, 156, 158t
in incidence of sarcoidosis, 38, 39t, 41t
in lupus pernio, 107t
in osseous sarcoidosis, 135t, 136
Radioactive scans, in evaluation of sarcoid
activity, 195–196, 195
Radiotherapy, in treatment of sarcoidosis,
230–231
Renal function tests, 170
Respiratory tract, sarcoidosis of, 49–76. See
also *Intrathoracic sarcoidosis, Pulmonary
sarcoidosis,* and *Upper respiratory tract.*
upper. See *Upper respiratory tract.*
Retinal sarcoidosis, 83
fluorescein angiogram of, 84
Rheumatism, acute, vs. arthralgia preceding
erythema nodosum, 142t
Rheumatoid nodule, 211, 212

Salivary glands, biopsy of, 33
Sarcoid granuloma(s), histology of, 21, 22, 23
metabolic formation of, 22
necrotising, differential diagnosis of, 61t,
67
progression to fibrosis of, 26–27, 27–29
Sarcoidosis, acute vs. chronic, differentiating
features in, 18t
aetiology of, 216–221
suspected factors in, 217t
biochemistry of, 163–173
clinical features of, comparative frequency
of, 39t

Sarcoidosis (*Continued*)
clinical features of, worldwide vs. Eastern Europe, 237t
clinical management of, recommendations for, 44
complications of, 48t
course of, 45–48
criteria of activity in, 192–198, 193t
clinical and bedside techniques for, 192
descriptive definition of, 17
differential diagnosis of, 199–215
epidemiology of, 233–246
familial, 243–244
first published account of, 1, *4*
granulomatous lung diseases and, differential diagnosis of, 60–68, 61t
historical background of, 1–16. See also *History, of sarcoidosis.*
malignant tumours and, 126–127
modes of presentation of, 40t
multisystem, clinical features of, 38–48
vs. local sarcoid-tissue reactions, 20t
ocular, 77–89. See also *Ocular sarcoidosis* and names of specific disease entities, such as *Uveitis.*
of alimentary tract, 144–155. See also specific organs.
of upper respiratory tract, 68–75. See also *Upper respiratory tract.*
paediatric, 155–160. See also *Childhood, sarcoidosis of.*
pathology of, 21–37
prognosis of, 45–48
index for, 45t, 46t
pulmonary. See *Pulmonary sarcoidosis.*
tissue markers in, 196t
tissues involved in, comparative frequency of, 39t
treatment of, 222–232. See also *Treatment, of sarcoidosis.*
world conferences on, 10–15, 11t, *11–13, 15*
Scars, 109–111, *110*
Schaumann's bodies, 24–25, *25*
Schistosoma, infective granulomas due to, 202
Schistosomiasis, in differential diagnosis, 202
lymphadenopathy in, 124
Scleritis, 85
Serological markers, in evaluation of sarcoidosis, 196, 196t
Sex, distribution of, in incidence of sarcoidosis, 38, 39t, 41t
in cardiac sarcoidosis, 114t
in childhood sarcoidosis, 156, 158t
in lupus pernio, 107t
Silica, granulomatous lymph nodes and, 127
Silicone, lymphadenopathy due to, 130, *130*
Silicosis, vs. pulmonary sarcoidosis, 62
Sjögren-like syndrome, 88, *88*

Skin, sarcoidosis of, 97–111
lesions of, 43
chronic, *138*
first patient with, 3, *3*
in upper respiratory tract sarcoidosis, 72
incidence of, 97t, 98t
treatment of, 225–227
Skin biopsy, 31
Skin tests, development of sarcoid granuloma in, 181t. See also *Kveim-Siltzbach skin test.*
Sodium cellulose phosphate, in treatment of sarcoidosis, 231
South Africa, incidence of sarcoidosis in, 233–235
Sperm granulomas, 209, *211*
Spirochaetes, infective granulomas due to, 200t, 202
Spleen, 118–119
aspiration biopsy of, 32
Splenomegaly, 118
Sporotrichosis, clinical features of, 201t
Starch, glove powder, granulomas due to, 154, *154*
Steroids, in treatment of sarcoidosis, 222, 223t
Stomach, 152–153
Syphilis, in differential diagnosis, 202
lymphadenopathy in, 123–124

T lymphocytes, abnormal activity of, 174
Talc, gastrointestinal granuloma due to, 154, *155*
lymphadenopathy and, 128
pulmonary granulomatosis due to, vs. sarcoidosis, 62, *63*
Tattoo granulomas, 211
Tenneson, 5
Thallium-201 imaging, in cardiac sarcoidosis, 116
in evaluation of sarcoid activity, 196
Tissue markers, in sarcoidosis, 196t
Toes, deformities of, in osseous sarcoidosis, 136, *137*
Tomography, positron, in pulmonary sarcoidosis, 59
Toxocara, infective granulomas due to, 200–202, 200t
infestation with, management outline for, 149t
Toxoplasmosis, and sarcoidosis, 218
in differential diagnosis, 200
lymphadenopathy in, 124, *124*
Treatment, of sarcoidosis, 222–232
criteria of cure in, 222t
drug regimens in, 223t
frequency of oral steroid use in, 223t
ineffective and harmful, 232

Treponema pallidum, lymphadenopathy associated with, 123
Tuberculosis, exposure to, relationship to
sarcoidosis of, 238, 240t
geographical regions of, 206t
in differential diagnosis, 202
lymph node granulomas in, 119
histological appearance of, *122*
management outline for, 149t
tests for, 206t
vs. sarcoidosis, 216–217
distinguishing features of, 203t
of upper respiratory tract, 74t
Tumours, in differential diagnosis, 205–208
malignant, sarcoidosis and, 126–127

United States, incidence of sarcoidosis in, 233
Upper respiratory tract, sarcoidosis of, 68–75
biopsy of, 34
chest radiographic changes in, 73t
chronic progressive, 74t
clinical features of, 42, 69t
course of, 73–75
differential diagnosis of, 74t, 75
intrathoracic involvement in, 72, 73t
multisystem involvement in, 72–73
ocular involvement in, 72
sites involved in, 69–71, 70t
skin lesions in, 72
treatment of, 225
Uric acid, levels of, 170, 171t

Uveitis, sarcoid, acute vs. chronic, age distribution in, *81*
anterior, 80
chronic, 89, *89*
posterior, 81
Uveoparotitis, historical background of, 9

Virus, as cause of sarcoidosis, 217

Wegener's granulomatosis, differential diagnosis of, 61t, 67, *68*
vs. sarcoidosis of upper respiratory tract,
74t
Whipple's disease, alimentary tract granulomas in, 155
lymph node granulomas in, 128
vs. sarcoidosis, differential diagnosis of,
156t
Willan, Robert, description of erythema nodosum by, 7

Yersinia, granulomas due to, 204
lymphadenitis associated with, 122–123

Zirconium, as cause of sarcoidosis, 219
Zirconium skin test, 180, 181t

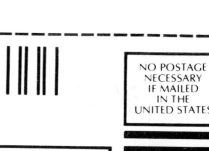